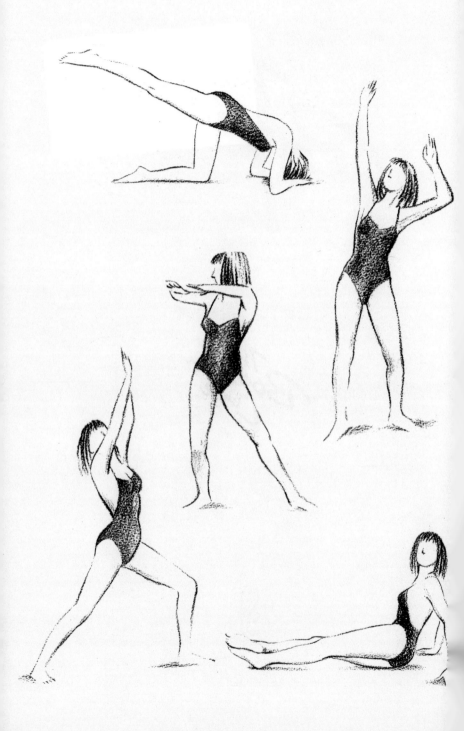

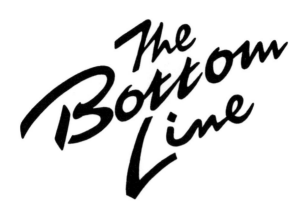

The Bottom Line

The Battle Against
Cellulite

Diana Moran

Foreword by Rosemary Conley
Facts and Figures by Elancyl

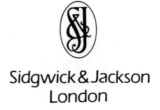

Sidgwick & Jackson
London

First published in Great Britain in 1989
by Sidgwick & Jackson Limited

Copyright © 1989 by Diana Moran

Line drawings by Paul Demeyer
Design by Paul Watkins

The author and publisher are grateful to Viking for
permission to use the diet devised by Nevil von Stenberg
which appears on p. 69, taken from
The Vogue Book of Diet and Exercise, and to the
Health Education Authority for permission to use
the weight chart which appears on p. 78.

ISBN 0-283-99804-0

Photoset by Rowland Phototypesetting Limited
Bury St Edmunds, Suffolk

Printed in Great Britain by
Butler and Tanner Limited
Frome, Somerset
for Sidgwick & Jackson Limited
1 Tavistock Chambers, Bloomsbury Way
London WC1A 2SG

Contents

Foreword
by Rosemary Conley

Anyone who says there's no such thing as cellulite has obviously never had to tolerate it. At last, here is a book that tells us what it is, why we get it and what we can do to get rid of it. And who better to tell us than the 'Green Goddess' herself – Diana Moran.

I can remember seeing Diana on television for the first time and hating her because she looked so fabulous. She had the sort of shape that I (and I'm sure many others) had always dreamed of. Diana was one of the first to put fun into fitness and the keep-fit fraternity has never looked back.

I had the pleasure of meeting and working with her for the first time last year. My initial fear and trepidation at meeting this very impressive lady was soon dispelled. Diana is a genuinely charming and friendly person, who wants everyone to feel relaxed, happy and healthy. She succeeds. So she is the perfect person to teach us how to make the most of ourselves.

The Bottom Line goes into a great deal of detail as to the facts about cellulite, but it does more than that. After all, what's the point of solving the cellulite if the rest of us isn't right? Diana has combined advice on exercise (of course!), on eating healthily, and on how to make the most of ourselves using fabrics and fashions to flatter. This is a book we've been waiting for for years.

Part 1

What is Cellulite?

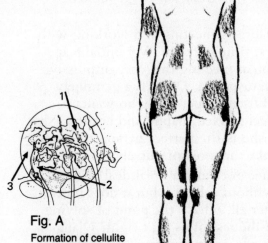

Fig. A

Formation of cellulite
1 Accumulation of
   water, toxins and
   fatty substances
2 Poor circulation
3 Ageing of connective
   tissue

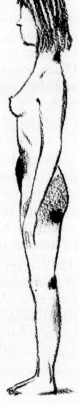

Fig. B

Understanding Cellulite

In my experience of over twenty years in the world of exercise, health and beauty, I have become increasingly aware as the years go by of a problem which affects many women. There is always at least one letter in my post-bag from a lady seeking advice on how to deal with the ugly dimpled skin which she has found on her bottom and which she has failed to shift even after slimming. Back in the 1920s, French beauticians gave this unsightly accumulation of fat-puckered skin a label which has since been adopted world-wide: cellulite.

But what exactly is cellulite and how is it formed? It has to do with our hormonal make-up (this is the reason why women suffer and not men) and is thought to be caused by a retention of excess fluid, and the accumulation of excess fat. The combination of fats, water and toxins trapped in the connective skin tissue results in a lumpy, dimpled look (see **Fig. A**) which gives the skin the appearance of orange peel. Cellulite can appear on women's thighs, hips, stomachs and sometimes their under-arms and knees (see **Fig. B**) and, although it is not unhealthy as such, it does not look very attractive.

Whatever British doctors may say, to the majority of women cellulite and obesity are not the same thing. In obesity the fat is spongy and flabby but smooth and no pain is felt when it's touched. Cellulite takes different forms but can be recognized, firstly, by the orange peel appearance of the skin (particularly noticeable when the muscles are contracted) and, secondly, if you can see the mark of your thumb after pressing the cellulite area (which may hurt when pinched). The condition can be triggered by a number of things, ranging from poor diet to lack of exercise. Certain

9

women – those who accumulate fat in the bottom/hip/thigh area – are more prone to it than others.

Cellulite is not, however, to be confused with cellulitis, the medical term for an inflammation of the skin which gives it a hard red shiny appearance.

In fact, in English-speaking countries we have been rather slow in facing up to the facts about cellulite: it would appear that continental ladies and their doctors (in France and Italy, in particular) have been aware of and trying to eliminate the unsightly flesh resulting from cellulite for many years. On the whole, however, most women were not bothered by the condition until the early part of the twentieth century since their flesh had hitherto been kept under wraps. A little flesh in the form of the shapely leg was revealed in the roaring 1920s and then even more with the birth of the mini skirt in the 1960s. The hip line became important with the advent of the trouser suit in the 1960s and 1970s. But it was the revival of jeans, designed to hug the figure like never before, at this time which made women of all ages conscious of their bottoms and thighs. Attempts to improve their bottom lines through exercise and diet often proved successful but still the quality of skin in this area caused many women distress.

The relatively recent concern with the condition is reflected in the attitudes of women of different ages: ask a woman of sixty years or more about her cellulite and she will probably be confused and unsure of just what you're referring to. Upon further probing she may confirm the presence of unattractive dimpled skin on her bottom and thighs which she has accepted as being inevitable with the passing of years. By contrast, when a twenty-year-old woman is questioned about cellulite, she is well aware of the problem and ready to fight the onset of the condition which makes her figure look prematurely old. She's only too eager to eliminate the ugly granular dimpled skin and is determined to do all she can to hang on to her youthful beauty for as long as possible.

These days, the word cellulite is part of most modern women's vocabulary; yet at the same time its meaning is not well understood. Obesity, fat, extra calories, and cellulite are all terms people váguely associate with each other – and nearly everyone knows they require *some* effort to control. Before any improvement can be seen you may need to remodel the contours of your body, and fight the insidious cellulite that has attached itself to particular parts of the body. The battle of the bulge begins. To win the battle it helps to know the most effective weapons to use and that's what this book is all about: solving the problem of cellulite by showing the numerous ways in which you can beat it. All the methods I will discuss are aimed at assisting you, whatever your age, to attain the sleek, healthy body you desire, and in doing so, enabling you to look good and feel great.

Certain members of the British medical fraternity may deny the existence of cellulite, maintaining that it is not a real problem, but as many of us know all too well, it really does exist and it really is a problem. A theory in the 1970s equated cellulite fat with inflammation of tissue but this was denied by many physicians. Since then, there has been a closer look at the problem and more medical research has been undertaken. The findings of this research have been analysed and it is now thought that cellulite is the amassing of fat and water in the connective tissue.

So let's take a closer look at the physiology of cellulite. As we know, it accumulates on the bottoms, thighs and hips of women of all shapes and ages, not only the well rounded. Even the slimmest women can find areas of cellulite developing in specific areas of their bodies. It's an affliction which can occur at any time between the ages of fifteen and fifty and once it has taken a hold, many women tend to believe it will be there for ever.

Scientists in France, particularly at the Elancyl laboratories, working in collaboration with the University of Toulouse, in collaboration with research teams in Italy, the USA and the USSR, have been investigating cellulite for more than fifteen years, but despite this the exact reason for its formation *still* isn't crystal clear. However, there does appear to be a close connection between the formation of cellulite and the female physiology; research indicates that one cause may be hormonal – a relative excess of the female hormone oestrogen may result in the condition. At present there isn't a counterbalancing treatment available. But in the meantime, please don't give up and resign yourself to the presence of the unsightly condition. By re-assessing your diet, taking more exercise, learning the art of self-massage, undergoing salon treatment or treating yourself at home, you *can* help yourself. But first, let's find out a little more about the make-up of our skin.

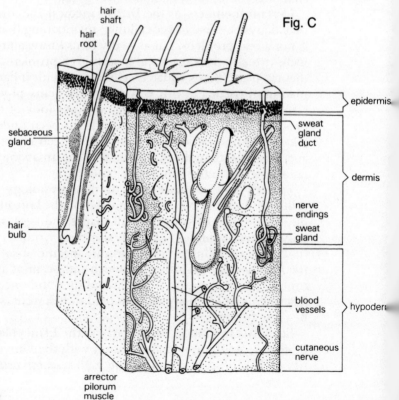

Fig. C

Getting to Know Your Skin

Unfair as it may seem, men generally seem to escape the problem of cellulite since their skin is arranged differently to ours and they have a different hormonal make-up.

To understand why many women are affected we must look more closely at the construction of our skin (**Fig. C**). It consists of three layers: the top layer, the epidermis, which is where the cells multiply and constantly renew themselves; it is also the protective layer. The middle layer, the dermis, consists of the connective and elastic tissues. These contain collagen and elastin, blood vessels, lymph and nerve endings. The connective fibres support and maintain the elasticity of the skin. The third, and deepest, layer of our skin, is the hypodermis. It contains the fatty cells and is the reserve tissue which gives the skin its suppleness. Since there is no wall between the dermis and the hypodermis, the fatty cells from the hypodermis are able to invade the dermis.

Both male and female skin have a hypodermic layer containing fatty cells. In female skin, however, these fatty cells have the ability to develop and multiply twice as quickly as in the male skin. An important factor to add to this is the sensitivity of the hypodermic layer to female hormones.

Now that we understand a bit more about the make-up of our skin, let's see where cellulite comes in. Cellulite is the abnormal accumulation of fat, toxins (found in coffee, tea, cigarettes and alcohol) and fluids deposited in the dermis. The fatty cells accumulate to form nodules, and collagen (a protein) then collects around the nodules which become trapped by the fibrous tissue. The more the collagen fibres surround

13

the nodules of fatty cells the more isolated they become. The blood capillaries around them become compressed which leads to bad circulation. Plasma is excreted creating an oedema (water retention) and an accumulation of toxins.

In more advanced cases of cellulite the collagen hardens. It is at this congested stage of the continuous process that the blood and lymph systems are rendered inefficient and unable to cope. The skin of the affected area becomes pitted and takes on the appearance of orange peel.

The Hormonal Influence

Hormones play an important part in the formation of cellulite. The female ovary secretes two hormones: oestrogen and progesterone. Both these hormones play crucial roles in a woman's menstrual and gestation cycle. Oestrogen causes water retention while progesterone helps to combat it. If all is well, the result is an equilibrium, or, to put it quite simply, a healthy balance. But if this balance is upset by a hormonal excess – for example a relative surfeit of oestrogen – then water, fat and toxic wastes are retained in the connective tissue. The whole situation is made worse if, in addition, you have poor circulation.

Each month during a woman's menstrual cycle, there are several natural fluctuations in the levels of female hormones. Seventy-five per cent of cellulite is seen to occur at the various stages of female sexual development and activity.

- **Twelve per cent** of cellulite, for example, is formed at puberty. In female adolescence, the ovary begins to function and at this time there is a total upheaval of all the hormones that will eventually transform the girlish figure into a womanly form. A glandular secretion secures the important production of oestrogen which is the essential female hormone. The young girl's body fills out; she loses her boyish hips, her breasts develop and the fatty tissue below the skin thickens.

- **Seventeen per cent** of cellulite forms during pregnancy. An excessive weight gain is all too often associated with pregnancy, but, fortunately, the old wives' tale of 'eating for two' has been dispelled as a myth and nowadays obstetricians keep a close watch on expectant mothers, recommending a balanced diet with lower weight gain. However, extra hormones are produced during pregnancy and these can cause water retention. Add to this bad circulation (the result of the baby pressing on the large veins of the abdomen) and cellulite is likely to form.

- **Twenty-seven per cent** of cellulite is formed premenopause. From about the age of forty onwards, the production level of oestrogen remains constant. However, the production of progesterone diminishes and the ensuing imbalance causes water retention. Gynaecologists can counteract this by prescribing progesterone treatment which restores the hormonal balance, thus slowing up the production of cellulite in women over the age of forty. The removal of the ovaries can also, of course, upset the hormonal balance.

- **Nineteen per cent** of cellulite occurs when oral contraceptives are taken. Some years ago, it was discovered that weight gain and the onset of cellulite was common in women when they started taking the pill, particularly the high-dose pill which was prescribed in the 1960s and 1970s. However, today's 'modern' pill, with its precise dosage and low oestrogen content means that the rise of water retention and the weight gain is far lower than it once was. Women who suffer from obesity and cellulite can take a progesterone only pill.

However, hormonal changes are not the only cause of fat cells forming. Let's take a look at the other factors that can assist and precipitate the accumulation of cellulite.

Circulation and Cellulite

Circulatory disorders are a problem and in some cases cause water retention in the tissues of the skin. This condition, known as oedema, occurs in the legs and ankles in particular. Women with bad circulation are prone to varicose veins and heavy legs, and many bruise easily. An unhealthy venous system can encourage the formation of cellulite.

A blocked circulatory system lessens the supply of oxygen to the tissues and it's worth mentioning here, as a word of caution, that this can be caused by tight elastic in socks, hold-up stockings, panties, girdles and bras. Jeans which fit too tightly around the waist, hips and thighs are also culprits and should be avoided. A larger size would be healthier and more comfortable too!

Sitting in any one position, standing, or even sitting with your legs crossed for too long are all bad for you as they impair lymphatic circulation and drainage thus encouraging the onset of cellulite. Women who lead sedentary lives – whether they work in offices, at factory benches or in front of machines all day – are therefore in danger! If our muscles are not exercised regularly and our circulation is not improved then cellulite *will* start creeping in, and, added to that, the infamous pear shape will be further accentuated.

Blood circulation in general and the venous system in particular benefit from physical exercise. Toning up the muscles of the stomach, bottom and legs in particular can help keep the body free of cellulite. The best way of doing this is by swimming or bicycling – both excellent forms of exercise for women of all ages and abilities. Swimming is particularly good exercise for those with heart problems or physical handicaps, since the body weight is supported by the water, thus facilitating exercise without over-exertion. Nevertheless, it is always wise to check with your doctor first if you do suffer from a heart problem, or have any other handicap, before going swimming. Exercise, whether on your own or in company, is beneficial. Gardening, jogging, team sport and brisk walking are all helpful.

Digestion and the Demon

A bad diet is another factor which can aid and abet the formation of cellulite. It is well known today that the Western diet is far from being a healthy one: in fact, it is recognized to be a killer. We generally consume too much fat, refined sugar and salt, which in turn can lead to weight gain (hence cellulite) and sometimes illness, like heart disease. So avoid foods which are rich in salt, fat and sugar, such as pastries, cakes and alcohol, and make sure you have plenty of fibre, in the form of fresh fruit, raw vegetables and wholegrain cereal for example. Fibre helps eliminate constipation and is a useful additive in any diet.

Part 2

Going into Battle

Facing up to Cellulite

Many women afflicted with a dense deposit of cellulite get upset about the condition; some even regard it almost as a physical handicap to such an extent that it affects them psychologically. The problem is compounded when help is sought from doctors, many of whom do not consider cellulite to be a medical problem. Private clinics are more sympathetic but often expensive and thus out of many women's range. There are health clubs and beauty salons that offer localized treatments using creams, gels and lotions combined with therapeutic massage and electrical treatment but these too can be expensive. There are also products you can buy for use in the privacy of your own home.

One thing to remember at all times, however, is that *you can beat cellulite*. In fact, not only can you eliminate it, you can also prevent its return with just the little time and effort required to fight the battle to its bitter end.

There are many, many forms of treatment available; some are more accessible than others, but all, I think, are worth a mention. The treatment you choose will depend on the type of woman you are and will reflect your age and lifestyle. Naturally, any anti-cellulite treatment is going to be a relatively short-term solution unless you use it in conjunction with a sensible diet and exercise programme. But I'll get to that a bit later.

Let's start with a closer look at massage which, for many years, has been the traditional way of helping to disperse cellulite, and remains one of the most effective techniques today.

Massage

The importance of massage in the battle against cellulite was recognized by the French laboratories Elancyl when in 1975 they developed a special glove to treat problem areas. The history of massage itself goes back thousands of years – as far back as the beautiful Egyptians, like Queen Nefertiti, who had their bodies regularly massaged with a pomade of roses, almond oil, honey and essential oils.

For the ancient Greeks and Romans, massage was an important method of relaxation and relief; Hippocrates in the fifth century BC swore by it; Julius Caesar, who suffered from neuralgia and migraines, often underwent massage to relieve his aches and pains. The essential and sweet smelling oils contributed to a feeling of well-being and sensuality.

Later on in history, the Arab physician Avicenna recommended massage to get rid of waste matter that settles in the muscles and cannot be got rid of through normal exercise. In France massage was used until the Middle Ages when religious taboos forbade its practice because of the pleasurable feelings it aroused. In the sixteenth and seventeenth centuries personal hygiene was not all it should have been and massage fell into disuse.

At the beginning of the nineteenth century a Swede, by the name of Per Henrik Lange, started what we today call **Swedish massage**. It was a mixture of gymnastics and massage techniques gleaned from the Chinese, Egyptians, Greeks and Romans, and introduced many of the terms now common in massage vocabulary, such as rolling, slapping, vibration, pinching and effleurage (meaning 'to skim over').

Swedish massage, the original classic movement, is both medically sound and therapeutic. It manipulates the muscles causing the blood, filled with toxins, to rise towards the skin where it throws off the toxins and becomes reoxygenated. The blood then returns to the organs, cleansed and regenerated. Medical massage had been born.

Shiatsu from the East is another popular form of massage and is the Japanese name for a type of massage that actually originated in China. It is based on acupuncture and uses acupressure – a form of acupuncture using the fingers – which stimulates reflex points. It works by pressing the fingers along the body's 'meridians' where the energy flows from head to foot.

Californian massage was invented at the Essalen Centre at Big Sur in California. It evolved from the experiences the Centre had had with the psycho-physical treatment of patients. Experts in this sort of massage consider it to be above all a sensual experience, both mentally and physically, and insist on the masseur and the patient building up a good rapport.

Lymphatic drainage is another form of massage which works on the lymphatic system. The lymphatic system, like that of the arteries and veins, is a drainage system for the body. Lymphatic drainage prevents the stagnation of the system. It consists of light rhythmic pummelling and pressure on the patient's back. These movements cause the lymphatic system to speed up and throw off its debris in a more efficient manner. The circulation is also improved and results are especially noticeable in cases where there is a lot of oedema in the cellulite-ridden areas.

Massage has several beneficial effects upon the body: the gentle friction created by rubbing the hands over the skin causes the blood vessels nearest the skin's surface to dilate which helps the blood to circulate; it speeds up the circulation and the function of the lymphatic glands which encourages them to throw off toxins; it helps make the connective skin tissues of the body more supple; it calms the nervous system, relaxes the body and helps smooth the dimply cellulite areas; it firms up the tissues of the skin and speeds up biological changes by the continuous stimulation of the cells.

Over the centuries massage has been proven, without a doubt, to be of tremendous benefit to the body by helping the nervous system and generating chemical changes. It also assists in maintaining the tone and shape of the body by encouraging women to feel and look good.

But not everyone has the opportunity, time or finances to take advantage of the skills of professional masseurs. Don't forget that in your own home you could equip yourself with the special **massage glove** designed to help combat cellulite by stimulating circulation and breaking down the nodular fatty areas. This treatment is completed with the application of a toning cream or gel.

There's no need to go to a salon either for this highly effective form of massage. When you have a bath try a **salt scrub**. Mix one tablespoon of sea salt and one tablespoon of kelp (available at good chemists) and massage into the cellulite areas, ideally using a loofah. Then rinse with warm water. Kelp is reputed to help diminish water retention, and the salt should improve the skin texture and stimulate blood flow to the area. Using sweeping strokes, you should work from the ankles up to the thighs, over the bottom and then, using small circular strokes, work up over the stomach towards the heart.

Increasingly, today's active woman is looking for methods of helping herself to improve her body in the privacy of her own home. With this in mind, cosmetic manufacturers, doctors and researchers have been working on products and methods for the modern woman which are both practical and effective.

Topical Treatments

Take a look along the shelves of good chemists and department stores and you will see a number of creams and gels designed to diminish localized cellulite areas. But just how effective are they?

In fairness to the manufacturers, these products are not meant to help with general weight loss but are specifically designed to attack areas of cellulite, such as the bottom, hips and thighs – areas which are difficult to improve with general dieting. The products show varying degrees of success in the battle against cellulite. A large proportion of women see the problem areas diminish – some more than others – but most see the skin becoming more firm and smooth.

In contrast to dieting aids, anti-cellulite products do not upset the body's equilibrium, nor do they cause tiredness or lack of energy. They work on localized areas, improving the look and feel of the skin. Used according to the manufacturers' instructions, they can, for many women, prevent the cellulite from returning. The modern woman demands efficient beauty aids that deliver good results and a great deal of cosmetic research is being undertaken in the laboratories to provide her with just that. Products are now available to help her attack fat, improve circulation and prevent premature ageing of the skin. The textures of these products are light and the thinking behind them sophisticated but, as we are well aware, women differ greatly in their requirements. Skin types, allergies, convenience, time and even moods must all be catered for. The result can be seen in the extensive variety of gels, creams and lotions which pander to our every need. But the effectiveness of any one product not only depends on its contents but also on its correct application and usage.

When we take a closer look at the anti-cellulite products we find that they fall into five categories:

Creams

These have a slow rate of penetration and will be favoured by women who regularly massage their body and faces with beauty creams. All massage is beneficial since it improves the circulation and tone of the body while only taking a few minutes of one's time.

Gels

These have been more recently formulated and are more quickly absorbed and less oily than the creams. When applied correctly they are very easily spread and don't leave the skin feeling sticky. The quick and easy application of these gels is particularly attractive to active, dynamic women with little time to pamper themselves.

As a result of intensive scientific research over the past few years, Elancyl technology has come up with the very latest thing: a gelled emulsion containing tiny particles which, when massaged gently into the skin with the finger tips, releases various active ingredients that are absorbed into the skin and help impart suppleness, improve the circulation and shift the deposits of fat. It takes hardly any time to apply and would appear to have long-term benefits.

Thermal Creams

Some women like to see instant results. They will be attracted to the thermal creams which improve the circulation through the heat caused by the properties of the cream. However, women with sensitive or fragile skins need to take care when using these.

Lotions

These products are for the woman in a hurry. They are convenient to use and easily absorbed by the skin.

Sun Creams

These use the heat of the sun to cause sweating which in turn expels water and toxins from the body. These products contain sun filters which allow safe tanning and spot reducing at the same time. Obviously they are only effective in hot weather.

The active ingredients in all the successful creams, gels and lotions are principally biological extracts of plants and seaweed plus vitamins. To be completely efficient they should be used in conjunction with other products by the same manufacturer.

The active ingredients in the products can be put into five important categories:

Lipolytics
The lipolytics dissolve fat. Peppermint tea is a good example. It attacks the fatty nodules trapped in the skin directly transforming them into fatty acids. These then escape through the layer of cellular membrane and are absorbed into the circulatory system.

Veinotonics
The veinotonics act on the blood vessels to get the blood moving. An extract of Ruscus (or Butcher's Broom – a prickly evergreen shrub formerly used for making brooms) assists the circulation by strengthening the blood vessels and accelerating the blood's passage through the veins and capillaries, often squashed by the cellulite. Ruscus has a stimulating effect on the lymphatic system, firming and improving its circulation and the drainage of toxins. It prevents the seepage of water into the tissues and makes better use of oxygen and nutritive substances. Hamamelis, red vine and horse chestnut are also used in medicinal concoctions to aid the circulation of the blood.

De-congestants and Filters
These ensure the efficient elimination of water and toxins, and ivy is at the top of this list, acting as a vaso-

constrictor (an agent which narrows the blood vessels) causing the blood capillaries to contract. It also works on the blood trapped in the cellulite areas and assists the blood flow to the heart ensuring a more efficient elimination of water and toxins. The extract of ivy's vitamin properties protect the circulatory system and its analgesic (pain relieving) properties help in relaxation. The ivy helps to dull the pain of cellulite which can be felt under pressure due to the compression of the nerve fibres. Meadowsweet (a fragrant flowering plant) is also used for its drainage properties.

Restructuring Agents
Having launched an attack on your cellulite, the skin in the problem areas needs help. The Elancyl laboratories were the first to recognize the crucial role Vitamin E could play here. Popularly known as the 'anti-ageing vitamin', it is claimed to stop the degeneration of the structure of the skin and help prevent the reforming and recurrence of cellulite as well as improving skin tone.

Let's take a closer look at how this works: oxygen is carried in the blood and oxidizes the different constituents of living matter. When this reaction is incomplete, toxic particles found in the body and in the air around us and known as 'free radicals' are released abruptly from certain molecules. These attack the skin cells, assault the connective tissue and weaken the collagen and elastin cells. These free radicals play an important role in the ageing process of our skin.

Vitamin E has an anti-oxidant effect on the substances in the body (it is oxidation which causes the skin to age); it can also improve the oxygen circulation in the blood. It prevents the formation of these free radicals and this in turn prevents tissue degeneration.

Firming Agents
Extracts from plants help firm and hydrate the skin. Horse-tail is rich in trace elements (iron and zinc), minerals and chemical catalysts necessary for the gen-

eral healthy functioning of the body. Along with birch, it has properties to firm and tone the skin.

Seaweeds are also rich in trace elements, vitamins and amino acids. Their properties also soften and hydrate the skin.

Application

To have any chance of effectiveness and success all these products must be used properly. The success of any treatment will depend almost wholly on the regularity and frequency of its use.

The products should mostly be applied once or twice a day for at least a fortnight, following the manufacturers' instructions, and then at regular intervals to prevent the return of cellulite.

The best time for application is after a warm bath when the skin is soft and can more readily absorb the creams, lotions and gels. Only a few minutes are required to apply them but a little pampering of the body helps to improve the texture of the skin and can also help in general relaxation. The pleasurable mixture of a relaxing bath and a soothing massage also goes a long way towards relieving stress.

To be able to relax is essential to our health and well-being. But many people at various times of their life find this very difficult. Psychological disorders, such as anxiety, anguish, nervous depression, over-emotion and stress, can result in people becoming addicted to the wrong sorts of food, such as junk food or chocolate, and thus lead to weight gain and the onset of cellulite. But stress need not be a twentieth-century hazard and the consequence of fast living if you think of yourself, and take time out to relax; make it a part of your daily routine to pamper yourself and your body.

Other Ideas

There is a whole range of other treatments for cellulite to be found in beauty salons, clinics and thalasso-therapy centres (centres specializing in treatments using water).

One particular form of **thalassotherapy** treatment consists of a whirlpool bath in which one soaks in water with active ingredients (seaweed and ivy) containing decongesting and filtering properties which act on the cellulite.

Iontophoresis is a treatment whereby ions of various soluble salts are introduced into the tissues by means of a constant electrical current.

Yet another treatment uses **infra-red rays**. The body is covered in a slimming product such as seaweed or ivy then enveloped in cling film. Then, on a sun bed the infra-red rays help in the absorption of beneficial properties of the plants.

Pressotherapy takes the form of an inflatable pair of trousers with double walls. These trousers put pressure on the cellulite tissues and help drain out the toxins.

During **laser treatment**, a cold laser of helium neon or infra-red is used to stop tissue hardening and to help relieve the possible pain of cellulite caused by the irritation of nerve fibres. It stimulates the cells and reduces the oedema.

Passive muscle exercise done with the aid of sophisticated electronic equipment works specific muscles without tiring the body out and is an alternative for people who do not like gymnastics.

Mesotherapy is a medical treatment which consists of hypodermic injections of active ingredients which diffuse through the skin to treat it.

Surgery is available for extreme cases. The following two operations are performed under general anaesthetic:

Liposuction: this consists of making an incision of about two centimetres in the skin into which is inserted a cannula (hollow tube). This sucks out the fat from the problem area. Many doctors are reluctant to recommend this method of treatment and it should only ever be performed by a competent practitioner.

Plastic surgery: this involves treating cellulite by the removal of fatty deposits on the stomach and the thighs through an incision in the skin. The skin is then carefully sewn up and after a few months the scar is hardly visible.

Measuring the Success of Your Treatment

Before the first *concrete* results in the battle against cellulite are to be observed a distinct improvement in the treated areas of skin cannot fail to be noticed; it starts to look more soft and silky and the texture becomes firm and supple. Gradually, as the treatment is continued, you should be able to see a distinct reduction of cellulite in the areas under attack.

As well as effectively combating the stubborn and unsightly cellulite, many of the products hydrate and nourish the skin thanks to the added vitamins, as we have seen. These penetrate deep down into the skin revitalizing the cells and helping the skin regain some of its lost elasticity. Manufacturers of the latest prod-

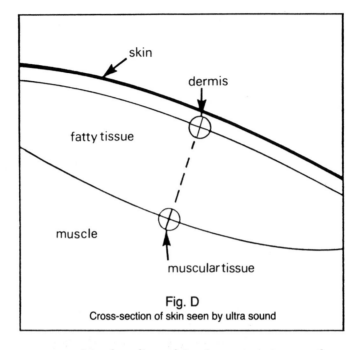

Fig. D
Cross-section of skin seen by ultra sound

uct, mentioned earlier, claim its properties can firm the skin and help fight against its ageing.

Of course, one may well be left asking: how effective are all these anti-cellulite products?

In recent years many clinical tests have been carried out in medical centres and hospitals, including the University Hospital in Toulouse, France. Several hundreds of women of all shapes, sizes and ages were tested with varying degrees of success but before analysis the actual state of the conjunctive tissue could only be guessed at.

However, thanks to modern technology, the precise infiltration of cellulite into the conjunctive tissue and its depth can now be monitored by a method called **echotomography**, which uses ultrasound to explore the subcutaneous layer of the skin. The ultrasound sends a signal reflecting any obstacle that it meets. The time taken for the echo to bounce back shows precisely the distance and thus the depth of the infiltrated tissue. The method is used over the cellulite area and the information is gathered and charted. A reading is taken before and after thirty days' treatment. The results are then monitored to provide an accurate assessment of the product's efficiency.

Another very reliable method of investigation is **thermography**. By using thermography, heat given off by different parts of the human body can be measured and correlated by the infra-red rays given off by the tissues. Normal skin tissue and tissue with cellulite maintain different temperatures – the area where cellulite forms tends to be warmer. At the start of the treatment these varying temperatures are mapped out on a thermal chart with different colours showing the areas with cellulite. At the end of the treatment another chart is prepared and it is possible to measure the change precisely by comparing the two charts, thus establishing the cellulite reduction.

Over the past two years, the Elancyl laboratories have conducted a survey backed up by clinical tests held in different regions of France, involving a cross-section of women. The survey was to gauge the effectiveness of their latest anti-cellulite product.

The area of cellulite to be treated on each woman was measured. Treatment involved the daily application of the gel containing micro-particles. After fifteen days' application, measurements were charted and a decrease of fatty tissue was noted. After a further fifteen days the routine was repeated and the physicians noted a further decrease. The treatment was then stopped and after fifteen more days the results showed a slowing down of the process, although an improvement in the skin tone was evident as a result of the continuing action of the Vitamin E in the micro-particles. Echotomography studies confirmed the positive results of the clinical studies. The average decrease in the areas of cellulite measured was three centimetres. As each woman was responsible for the application of the product herself, the human element may account for 20–25 per cent who failed the test.

All these methods of assessing the efficiency of anti-cellulite products are not, of course, available in the privacy of your own home. To test the effectiveness of whatever method of attack you have chosen you should measure the reduction of the specific areas of cellulite as they are treated. For example, the cellulite on a thigh should be measured before treatment and then again thirty days later and the difference noted.

The fight against cellulite is irritatingly difficult and one which needs perseverance if any improvement is to be noted. There is no magical cure for the resilient deposit but help is at hand with the new specialized products and massage appliances already mentioned. Results will only be seen, however, if the attack on the specialized areas is kept up. This requires both patience and determination as well as good general hygiene, an increase in exercise and a new, improved diet.

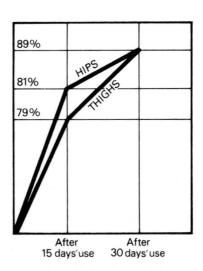

After   After
15 days' use   30 days' use

Fig. E
Results of supervised experiment
using anti-cellulite gel with microparticles

Part 3

Exercise

Any Time, Anywhere

Exercise alone will not make us lose weight but it *will* tone and firm the body that has not slimmed through the correct diet. We can help ourselves to better health by taking twenty minutes of exercise, ideally at least three times a week. This can take the form of sport, gardening, jogging or even a brisk walk, enough to raise the heart rate and make us feel a little puffed. Swimming is an excellent form of exercise for anyone of any ability; the handicapped too can benefit since the body weight is supported by the water.

I'm not going to suggest a rigid programme of physical exercise, as I believe it should be a pleasurable part of life and not a chore. Not everyone has the time or opportunity to take regular exercise in the form of a particular sport at a club, but this is not an excuse because some form of movement can be fitted into the busiest of schedules simply by exercising whenever and wherever an opportunity presents itself. Even in the car or at your desk you can pave the way to better posture, greater mobility and improved circulation and digestion by simple movement.

The secret of an improved lifestyle is self-motivation; without this all your good intentions will come to nothing. It's pointless to plan changes if the willpower isn't sufficient to get you up and out of your chair to take some positive action. Remaining glued to your seat for twelve hours a day and then spending the rest of your time in bed thinking about making changes is no good at all. A sedentary lifestyle encourages the slowing down of the body's metabolism.

You can begin by making small changes in your daily routine. Why not leave the car behind and walk to the station? Walk wherever possible, and use the stairs instead of lifts. Even when life is hectic at least spare the body a few minutes to stretch, just like a cat does on waking up! You can even stretch while still in bed in the morning. When you do get up simply reach for the ceiling then down to your toes. A few daily exercises will soon get you back into shape. So take every available opportunity to move a little in the kitchen, the garden, the office or even while waiting for the tube, bus or taxi. Here are some examples.

If you're waiting in a queue don't just move from one leg to the other, make the most of this time to exercise your muscles and oxygenate your blood: think about each muscle of your body beginning with your feet. Clench your toes, stretch the legs, stretch your back, lift your shoulders. Hold for a few seconds then relax your whole body and begin again. This will help relax your body and relieve the tensions of the day.

In the car, help yourself to relax by squeezing the steering wheel very tightly and breathing in at the same time. Hold for a few seconds, relax your hands and breathe out.

Sitting at your desk or work bench you can prevent back ache by doing the following exercises several times a day: stretch your arms high above you, fingers pointed towards the ceiling (**Fig. 1**). Breathe in and stretch your back out. Breathe out slowly, bring your arms down, bend your body forward and touch the floor (**Fig. 2**).

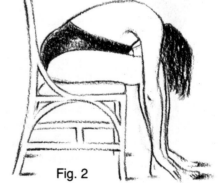

Fig. 1

Fig. 2

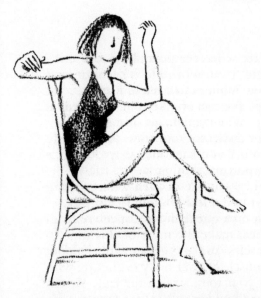

Sit well back in your chair and sit up straight. Breathe in, pull in your stomach muscles and push your waist into the back of the chair. Hold for several seconds, breathe out and relax the body. This simple movement repeated several times a day will help tone your stomach muscles and avoid an aching back.

Fig. 3

To improve circulation and digestion: sit forward in the chair, raise your right knee and touch it with your left elbow (**Fig. 3**). Repeat on the other side.

Fig. 4

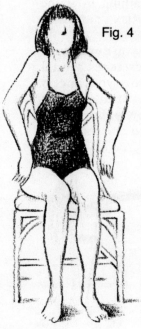

To release tension in the neck, shoulders and upper back whilst sitting or standing simply lift your shoulders up to your ears. (*Don't* lower the ears to the shoulders.) (**Fig. 4**)

Another simple exercise, again to release tension in the neck, shoulders and upper back, is to raise the shoulders up and forward (**Fig. 5**) then take them back down and around (as in the butterfly swimming movement).

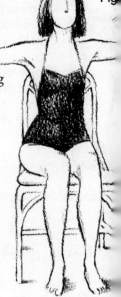

Fig

34

A simple exercise to relieve tired legs and feet can be done in front of the television at the end of a busy day. While seated lift and straighten one leg. Point the toes and keeping the leg still draw a circle with the toes (**Fig. 6**) exercising the ankle and foot, thus improving the circulation. Bad circulation, as we know, is one of the main contributing factors in the formation of cellulite. You can also improve the tone of your leg and thigh muscles: sitting in a chair place an object such as a cushion or waste paper basket between your ankles. Simply raise and lower both legs while holding the object tightly (**Fig. 7**).

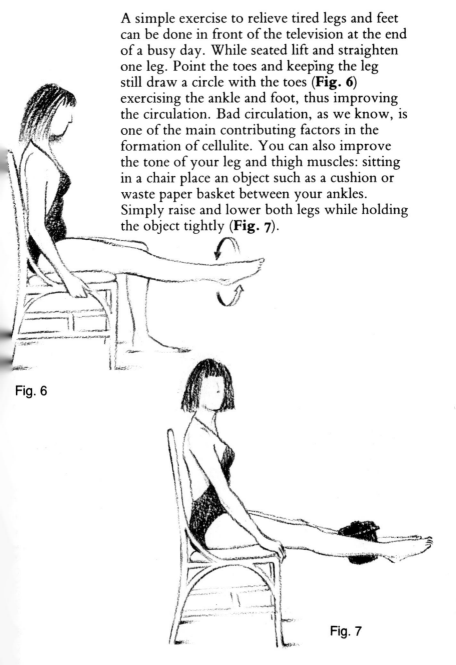

Fig. 6

Fig. 7

Too much sitting down can cause the muscles of the bottom and upper thigh to become lazy and flabby. So whenever you are standing, maybe cooking a meal or talking on the 'phone, you can still help yourself. Simply squeeze your bottom muscles together, hold for five seconds and relax. Repeat this as many times as possible.

Still standing, with your feet together, simply raise yourself up on to your toes (**Fig. 8**), working the thigh and bottom muscles, hold for five seconds and relax.

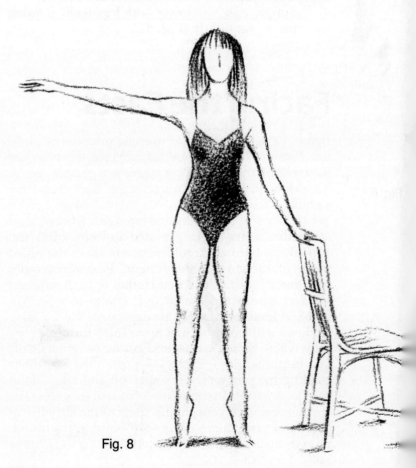

Fig. 8

And, at the end of a long day, learn to relax while taking your bath: lift your feet and rest them on the edge of the bath, place a towel under your neck and lean back. Before you get out of the bath use the hand shower. Make the most of the shower to massage your bottom with soap or gel with a circulatory movement. Spray the water from the ankles up to the thighs. Gradually day by day lower the temperature of the water. This tones the skin and protects it from the cold. If you are lucky enough to have a shower equipped with a massage fixture, use this with a circulatory movement on your legs, hips and bottom.

Facing the Facts

Before launching into a *full* exercise programme, let's just consider how our health is affected when we are overweight and unfit. First, there is a greater risk of high blood pressure and heart disease. We feel uncomfortable, short of breath and our circulation isn't good. We lack energy, mobility and strength. Rheumatism and arthritis may be aggravated and our joints feel stiff. Backs become a problem as a result of the added strain of carrying excess weight. Posture becomes bad, and it's difficult to find clothes to fit and flatter. We feel fed up and the circle is complete when we nibble at foods because we are depressed. We feel lazy, sit down and feel more and more sorry for ourselves.

So where should we begin? First we must get up off our bottoms, set ourselves a goal, then set about tackling the problem. Let's strip off and take a long hard look in the mirror. Many of us will see excess fat. If you press with your thumb some of the fatty flab at the top of your thighs or on your bottom, the thumb print remains. And if you pinch it between your thumb and index finger, it resembles the skin of an orange and might also be painful. These, as we know, are the three clinical signs of cellulite.

And while you're being so honest with yourself, take a good look at your back view too. Those hips and shapely thighs were built to carry and bear children. It's an area pre-disposed to fat and it contains large muscle masses. But if it's sat upon and the muscles aren't used enough they lose their tone. Thunder thighs and a broad beam may result. Add to this sluggish circulation and you can see how problems such as cellulite begin. The answer is to get it all moving again. Exercise can break down the fat by using it up as energy and not allowing it to be stored on the hips, thighs and stomach. With a mild work-out, exercise will stretch and tone the existing muscle mass and improve circulation. The aim is to not build more muscle but if this is required it can be achieved by using weights or resistance.

So it's time for action. But we must remember not to set ourselves too difficult a task. We're all made differently and bone structure, family traits and metabolism must all be taken into account. It's no good trying to be reed thin when our body type is large. So take it slowly, and if a particular movement hurts then leave it for today and try again tomorrow. The plan is to start slowly and build up gradually. Listen to your body, don't overdo things and, lastly, remember you're never too old or too young to start. A word of warning though to anyone who feels unwell, suffers from heart problems, obesity, a bad back or trouble with the joints: *take care* and, if in doubt, *consult your doctor* before contemplating an exercise programme.

The Real Benefits of Exercise

Learn to fit exercise into your day however busy you are and when there's a break in your work, literally take a breather and stretch. You'll revitalize your body, re-oxygenate your system and improve your circulation and digestion, all of which will help fight your cellulite and discourage its reappearance. Regular exercise, which should include some aerobic work such as exercising to music, jogging or skipping, will speed up our bodies' metabolic rate and help to burn up excess calories. Being fit adds quality to everyday life and if you work at it you will improve your chances of physical independence in later years. It will take two to three months before the real benefits of regular exercising are felt, but eventually it will increase our Suppleness, Stamina and Strength, the three 'S's of exercise. But there is a fourth 'S' – sex which improves when we look good and feel great.

Once you have achieved a certain level of fitness, you should think about moving on to join a sports club or a gymnasium, or perhaps take up martial arts. Go jogging or dig the garden and, in your spare time, walk or go dancing (even the disco can be good exercise). So make the effort and find a form of exercise to suit you. Through sport you can work out your frustrations and life becomes richer. But remember, you must get fit to keep fit!

A Twenty-Minute Session

Let's begin with a stretch . .

1 **Stand with feet shoulder width apart.**
2 **Stretch arms high above head (Fig. 9).**
3 **Bend the knees, swing arms down to the side and back behind (Fig. 10).**
4 **With a continuous movement, straighten knees, swing arms forward and up and reach for the ceiling.**

Repeat to warm up and stretch out the whole body.

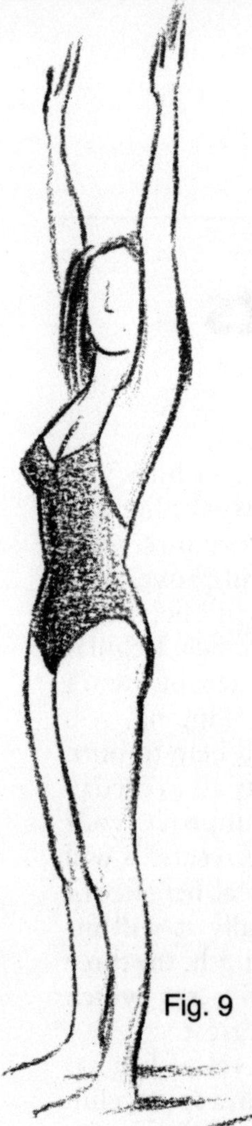

Fig. 9

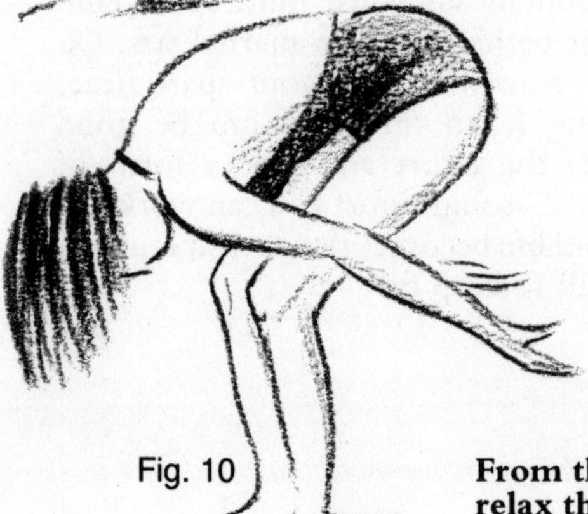

Fig. 10

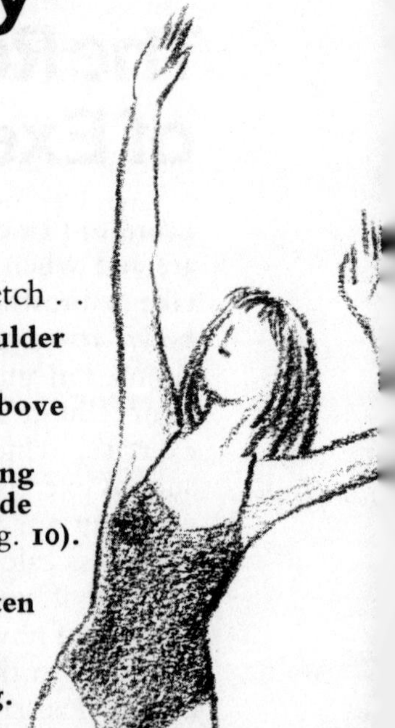

Fig. 11

From the same starting position, relax the knees and with alternate arms reach up as high as possible to stretch the sides of the body (Fig. 11).

1 Stand with feet further apart, arms up at shoulder level.
2 Twist *upper* body around to look first to the right side and then to the left (Fig. 12).

1 Stand with feet wider apart.
2 Turn left foot out and keep right foot straight ahead.
3 Bend left knee over left foot and twist upper body to face left.
4 Lift arms up high and push out to the left, working legs and stretching through the body (Fig. 13).
5 Keep both feet flat on the floor. Repeat with right side.

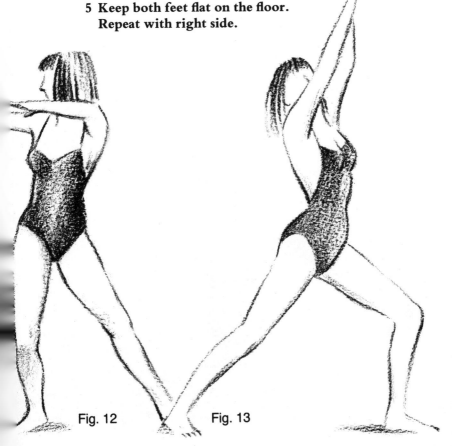

Fig. 12   Fig. 13

Now that you have mobilized your body with these simple movements it's time to concentrate on some exercises which will work specifically on the muscles of the legs and bottom, helping to tone and trim your thighs.

1 **Using a chair back or table top for support, stand with your heels together and knees turned out.**
2 **Bend the knees and, keeping a straight back, pull in the stomach muscles.**
3 **Bend the knees and lower down as far as comfortable (Fig. 14).**

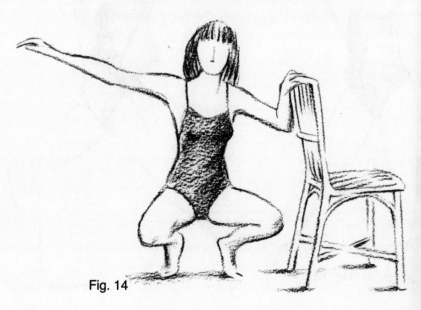

Fig. 14

1 Again use furniture for support, standing with feet twelve inches apart, toes and knees turned out.
2 Bend the knees, keep feet flat on the floor and lower down as before (Fig. 15).

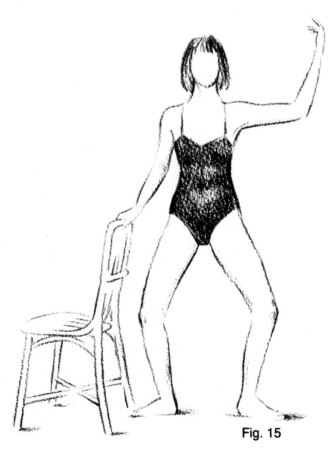

Fig. 15

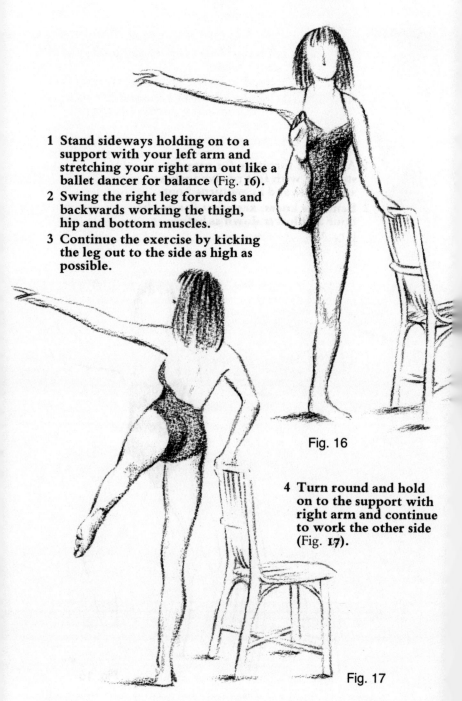

1 Stand sideways holding on to a
   support with your left arm and
   stretching your right arm out like a
   ballet dancer for balance (Fig. 16).
2 Swing the right leg forwards and
   backwards working the thigh,
   hip and bottom muscles.
3 Continue the exercise by kicking
   the leg out to the side as high as
   possible.

Fig. 16

4 Turn round and hold
   on to the support with
   right arm and continue
   to work the other side
   (Fig. 17).

Fig. 17

44

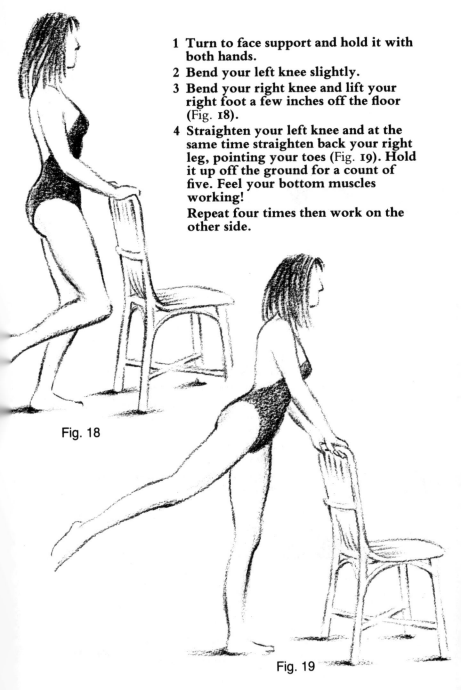

1 **Turn to face support and hold it with both hands.**
2 **Bend your left knee slightly.**
3 **Bend your right knee and lift your right foot a few inches off the floor (Fig. 18).**
4 **Straighten your left knee and at the same time straighten back your right leg, pointing your toes (Fig. 19). Hold it up off the ground for a count of five. Feel your bottom muscles working!**

Repeat four times then work on the other side.

Fig. 18

Fig. 19

45

Time now to get to the bottom of things with a few floor exercises to tighten and trim that bottom and strengthen your back at the same time. If, however, you suffer with back problems, do not attempt these exercises.

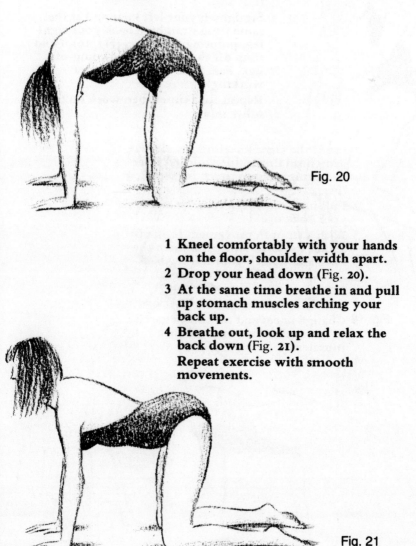

Fig. 20

1 **Kneel comfortably with your hands on the floor, shoulder width apart.**
2 **Drop your head down** (Fig. 20).
3 **At the same time breathe in and pull up stomach muscles arching your back up.**
4 **Breathe out, look up and relax the back down** (Fig. 21).
   Repeat exercise with smooth movements.

Fig. 21

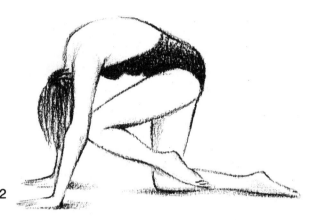

Fig. 22

1 From the same kneeling position
   drop head down, lift your left knee
   and bring it up to touch forehead
   (Fig. 22).
2 Pull in the stomach muscles and arch
   your back up.
3 With a smooth movement look up
   and at the same time straighten the
   knee and stretch your left leg back
   and up and hold for five seconds (Fig.
   23).
4 Gently return to the original position.
5 Change knees and continue exercise
   to strengthen bottom and back
   muscles.

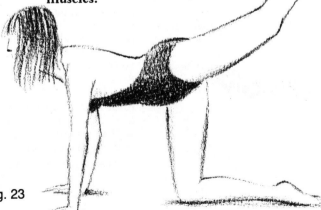

Fig. 23

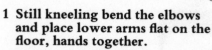

1 Still kneeling bend the elbows and place lower arms flat on the floor, hands together.
2 Bend forward and rest head on hands.
3 Pull up stomach muscles.
4 Lift and straighten right leg back parallel to floor (Fig. 24).
5 With a restrained movement bob the leg up and down to tone and tighten bottom and thigh.
6 Repeat with the left leg.

Fig. 24

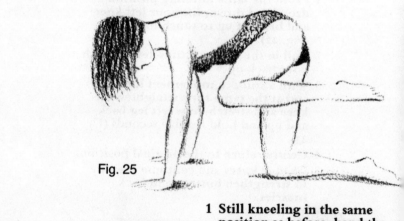

Fig. 25

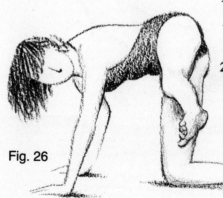

Fig. 26

1 Still kneeling in the same position as before, bend the left knee, taking it forward and out to the side parallel to the floor (Fig. 25).
2 Straighten out the leg, still keeping it parallel to the floor and pointing the toes (Fig. 26). This movement will work on the hip and thigh muscles.

Repeat with the other side.

48

1 **Still kneeling straighten the upper body.**
2 **Place your right hand on your right ankle.**
3 **Raise your left arm up and over to the right side, stretching your left side (Fig. 27).**
   Repeat the movement with the other side.

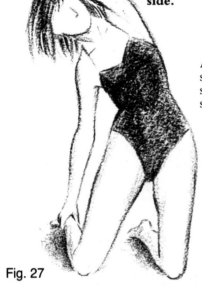

All exercises like this involving stretching are good because they stretch the connective tissue and stimulate lymphatic circulation.

Fig. 27

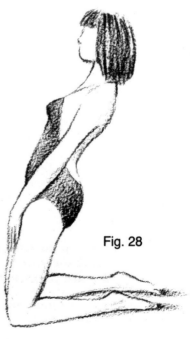

1 **Kneel up straight, arms at your side.**
2 **Gently move your upper body backwards controlling the movement with thigh and bottom muscles (Fig. 28).**
3 **Hold for five seconds and return gently to the original position.**

Fig. 28

Sit on your 'seat' while you continue to work on your bottom and also your stomach muscles.

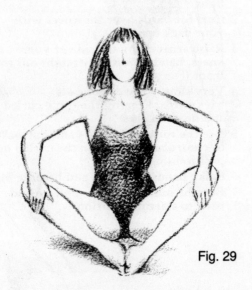

Fig. 29

1 **Sit on the floor with your knees bent and the soles of your feet together.**
2 **Place your hands on your knees and gently rock from side to side controlling the movement with the bottom and stomach muscles (Fig. 29).**

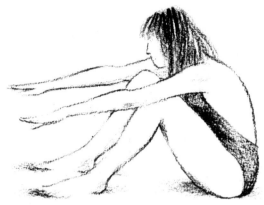

Fig. 30

1 Sit with knees bent and feet flat on floor.
2 Curl forwards over the knees with your back bent.
3 Raise arms up by the side of your knees, hands pointing straight out to front (Fig. 30).
4 Very slowly lower yourself backwards, keeping the spine curled and head on chest.
5 Use the tummy muscles and buttocks to control and maintain the curled up position (Fig. 31).
6 Relax hands on thighs and breathe in.
7 Breathe out and slowly pull up and back to starting position.

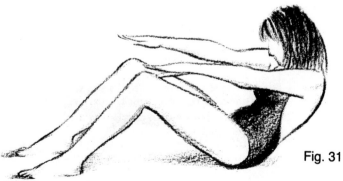

Fig. 31

51

Those of you with a weak back *can* do the following floor exercises which concentrate on turning your wobbles into wiggles by working on your hips, thighs and bottom – all the areas where cellulite is most likely to occur.

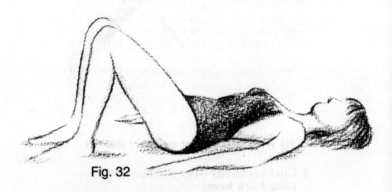

Fig. 32

1 **Lie back on the floor, arms at your sides, knees bent and feet shoulder width apart, flat on floor (Fig. 32).**
2 **Clench the buttocks, pull in the tummy and lift the pelvis up transferring your weight on to your shoulders (Fig. 33).**
3 **Hold for five seconds, relax and repeat.**

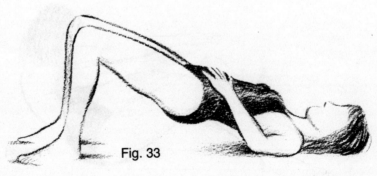

Fig. 33

1 Lie on your back, arms wide apart.
2 Pull your knees up to your chest (Fig. 34).
3 Twist from the waist and roll your knees over to the left side placing them on the floor.
4 Keep shoulders in contact with floor and face the right (Fig. 35).
5 Bring your knees back to the centre of your chest and roll them over to the right side. Now face the left.

This exercise will trim your bottom and middle and keep you supple.

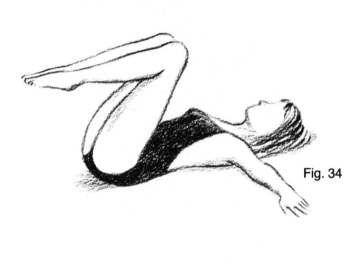

Fig. 34

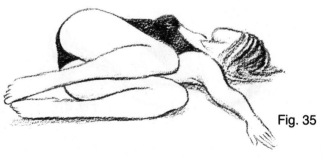

Fig. 35

1 Lie flat on the floor with your hands under your bottom.
2 Bend the knees outwards.
3 Bring your feet up and place soles together (Fig. 36).
4 Straighten legs up and out (Fig. 37). Repeat this exercise to strengthen inner thighs.

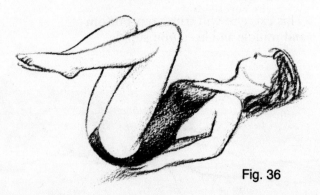

Fig. 36

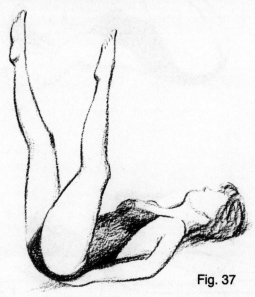

Fig. 37

1 **Lie on your left side and support the upper body on your left elbow.**
2 **Place your right hand on the floor in front of your waist for balance** (Fig. 38).
3 **Bend your right knee, touching your left knee with your right toes.**
4 **Straighten right leg up and point toe to ceiling** (Fig. 39).
   Repeat movement to strengthen and firm thighs. Turn over and repeat with the right side.

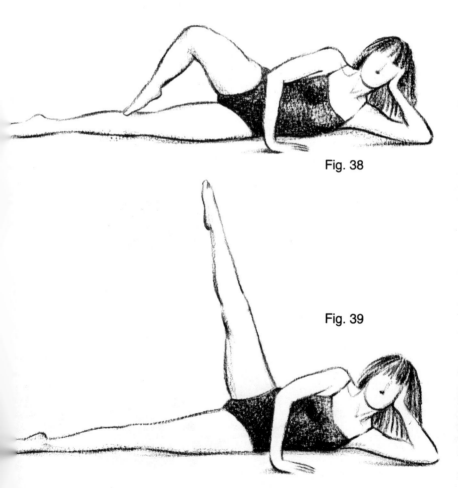

Fig. 38

Fig. 39

1 Lie on your left side supporting your
  head with your left hand, and with
  your right hand on the floor as
  before.
2 Raise your right leg up
  approximately twelve inches (Fig. 40).
3 Bring your left leg up to join it (Fig. 41).
4 Hold and squeeze your thighs, knees,
  calves and ankles together for a count
  of ten.
5 Relax and lower both legs.
  Roll over and repeat on the right side.

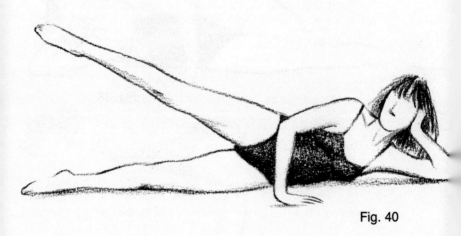

Fig. 40

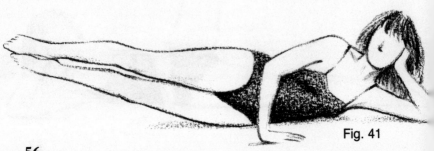

Fig. 41

These simple movements will, if done properly, make your seat neat (although they are not recommended if you suffer with a bad back).

1 **Lie on your stomach.**
2 **Turn your head and rest your cheek on your hands.**
3 **Keep your cheek in contact with your hands and lift both legs up (Fig. 42).**
4 **With feet flexed kick out to the sides.**
5 **Bring feet back together and repeat movement.**
 In the same position vary the movement by kicking the legs up and down with smaller scissor movements, keeping your hips on the floor (Fig. 43).

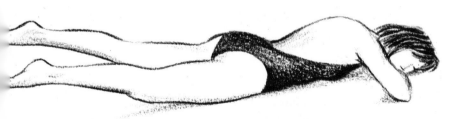

Fig. 42

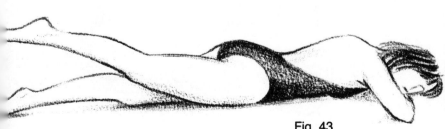

Fig. 43

57

These final floor exercises will firm and tone the bottom and entire leg. All exercise helps though in the fight against cellulite by improving circulation.

Sit up keeping back straight and stretch arms and legs out to the front. Aim to inch your way forwards by bending and lifting alternate legs, transferring weight from side to side, and using the bottom and stomach muscles (Fig. 44).

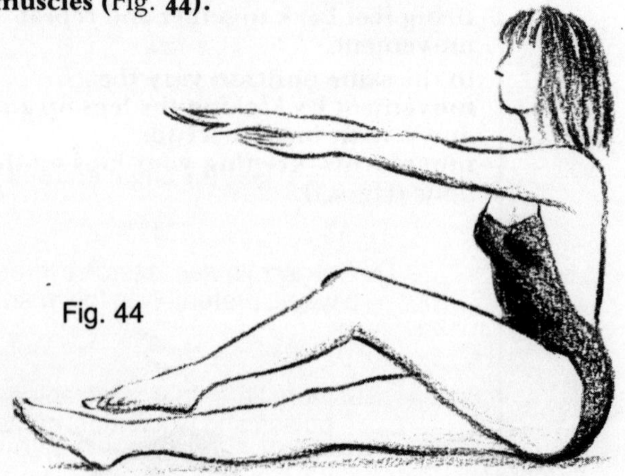

Fig. 44

1 **Lean back, placing your weight on your hands.**
2 **Cross your legs at the ankles.**
3 **Clench and lift your bottom, rocking and rolling from side to side (Fig. 45).**
  You deserve a rest – now lie back, relax your legs and arms and take a breather!

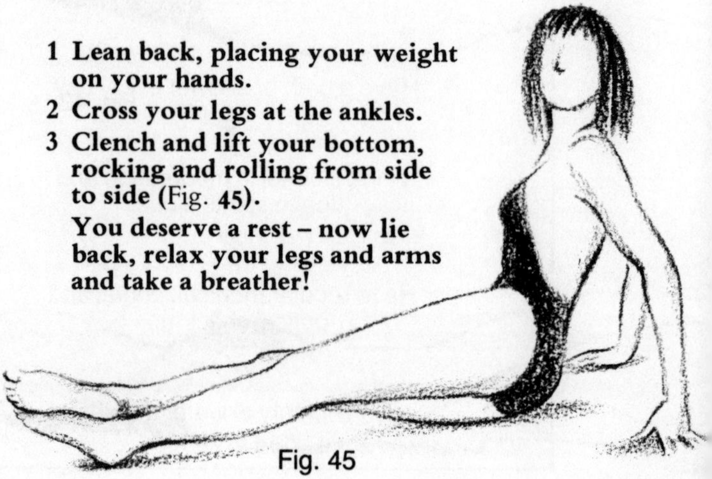

Fig. 45

Finally, remember – exercise alone is not enough. Bear in mind my ten basic tips for a healthy lifestyle which will keep you fit while at the same time helping to combat the dreaded cellulite:

Ten tips for a healthy lifestyle

Start each day with breakfast.

Stretch out your body each morning.

Eat less fat, sugar and salt.

Do twenty minutes' exercise three times
a week, preferably in the fresh air.

Eat more fibre, fruit, vegetables, nuts,
pulses and wholemeal bread.

Don't smoke.

Have a bath or shower every day.

Drink alcohol in moderation and
leave spirits alone.

Have regular medical, dental and
optical check-ups

Drink plenty of water to purify
your system.

Part 4

Diet

Getting the Healthy Habit

Good eating habits should be encouraged from an early age with confectionery, cakes and biscuits kept to a minimum. Fresh fruit should be substituted as treats. At puberty (average age thirteen) it is essential for young girls to be given guidance and advice to avoid unsightly 'puppy fat'. It should be noted that this is one of the peak times for the formation of cellulite. Good nutritional habits encouraged at this period of a girl's development are likely to become firm rules for a healthy adult life. A sensible eating pattern and a well-balanced diet should take the young adult through to maturity and will assist her in later years. It's never too late for the ill-informed or stubborn to reassess their lifestyle and to make healthy changes. The added years are no excuse for added inches. You can *never* be too old *or* too young to help yourself to better health.

First of all the body should be drained of existing waste matter that has accumulated through abusing our bodies. This takes the form of uric, lactic and oxalic acids. Overeating clogs up the system causing bodily malfunctions. The joints become stiff and the neglected overweight body functions inefficiently placing extra strain on the heart and lungs which in turn causes breathlessness. The digestive system is affected resulting in intestinal problems such as constipation.

With this increased understanding of just how we maltreat our bodies our fight against cellulite can continue. By now, we are aware of two important factors which cause changes in the conjunctive tissue of our skin. As we have previously discovered, the malfunction of a woman's hormones or a poor diet can cause an unnecessary weight gain. Now we must decide on a positive plan of action. If stage one in our battle was the use of anti-cellulite products combined with a regular exercise programme, then let stage two be a new, improved diet.

Shaping Up

Many of us are overweight and in being so we are doing ourselves a disservice, especially in the battle against cellulite. To lose weight and stay in shape is plain and simple common sense. Shedding excess weight improves general health and mobility and at the same time increases self-esteem. With a healthy body invariably goes a healthy mind and the ability to make the most of life. A slim woman often looks and feels years younger than her overweight friend.

Care must be taken, however, when choosing a method of weight control, since many can be harmful to one's health. Appetite suppressors, diuretics and calorie burners are not the long-term answer and should be used for short periods only, if at all. They may indeed result in a substantial weight loss during the first few weeks in which they are used, but they are dangerous on a long-term basis because they deny the body the valuable vitamins and minerals required for good health. They also have no effect on cellulite. Should there be a hormonal imbalance in the body, due to over-production of oestrogen, or a deficiency in progesterone which has encouraged the formation of cellulite, then this condition should be treated by a gynaecologist or endocrinologist.

Uncontrolled, very low calorie, diets should be avoided, since when weight is lost too quickly it is put back on again after the diet is finished. This can have an unbalancing effect on the body and can be dangerous.

A slower, more controlled weight loss should be aimed for.

While very low calorie diets are useful for some people with a lot of weight to lose, a complete re-assessment of eating habits is required to control cellulite and a *permanent* change should be made, not just a temporary one. The new-found habits should then become an integral part of your lifestyle.

In order to banish cellulite, a critical assessment of one's eating habits is essential: out go fats, refined sugar, excess salt and alcohol; in come lean meats, raw vegetables, skimmed milk and plenty of water and fresh fruit juices. The aim is to purify your body's system and rid it of excess toxins (the 'poisons' in the blood stream). An anti-cellulite diet may well help you to lose weight generally because you will find that you are consuming fewer calories.

Before I go any further let me explain just what a calorie is. A calorie is a measure of energy applied to food and drink. If we consume more calories (energy) than our bodies need for daily functioning and repair then the excess simply gets stored in our bodies and appears as unsightly fat.

To start with, therefore, your daily calorie intake should be noted. Your calorie count should include *everything*, not just the food consumed at meal times but all the nibbles snatched between meals and any liquid intake. Everything must be taken into account and all calories counted. Your total calorie intake should balance the calorie output of your body.

You must learn to kick your bad eating habits, however small and unimportant they may seem. That pang of hunger must be resisted and not satisfied by a biscuit, bar of chocolate, piece of cake or a sweet. If the desire to nibble between meals cannot be controlled then make the nibbles healthy ones: cut up and prepare vegetables containing very few calories and have them ready and easily accessible in the fridge to satisfy your cravings. Cucumber, celery, cauliflower and carrots are all easily prepared; they satisfy hunger pangs and have a beneficial and diuretic effect on the body.

If your impulse to nibble is very strong, help yourself by keeping temptation out of sight. Put your 'red light' foods in cupboards or up on high shelves. And store foods in the fridge in opaque containers so that you can't see the contents.

Don't do too much sampling while preparing and cooking meals. And, mums, don't become the family dustbin by eating the leftovers! Clear the table at the end of the meal and place the plates immediately into a sink full of soapy suds. While eating with the family fool yourself into thinking you're eating a large meal by serving your own helping on a small plate.

So what should you be looking for to improve your eating habits and how should you go about it? The mention of dieting and calorie counting can, I admit, be a boring turn-off, so a little imagination is called for.

Let's begin with the basics. Water, whether straight from the tap, or with added sparkle from a bottle, aids to speed up kidney activity and drinking up to six pints a day will be beneficial in controlling cellulite by flushing away toxins. So don't hinder this action by adding excess salt to your diet since this will only encourage water retention. Water can cleanse your system and can satisfy hunger pangs; a glass before your meal will make you feel full. Salt, by contrast, has neither of these beneficial effects.

Eat slowly and enjoy your food but don't overeat. I remember learning a lesson from my Victorian grandparents who taught me to leave the table feeling as if I'd like to eat just that little bit more. With work, activity and exercise your body should then use up all the calories in the food you have just eaten and also some of those already stored up as fat on your bottom. On high days and holidays you'll want to binge, so don't be a party pooper: go on and enjoy yourself but abstain the following day.

Set aside time for a good breakfast each day. Why

Anti-Cellulite Dietary Check List

Recommended	Not recommended
Fresh fruits (especially citrus)	Bananas
Vegetables (preferably eaten raw or lightly cooked)	Avocados
White meat	Red meat (unless trimmed of fat)
Fish	
Wholemeal bread	White bread
Bran cereal	
Potatoes (especially the skins)	
Low-fat cheeses	Hard cheeses
Skimmed milk	Cream
	Butter
Fruit and vegetable juices	Alcohol
Water	Tea
Herbal infusions (e.g. camomile)	Coffee
Yoghurt	
	Cakes and pastries
	Chocolate
	Sugar
Pulses	Peanuts
	Salt
	Processed foods (e.g. bacon, salami and anything canned or packaged)

not mix your own muesli (non-sweetened of course!) from wheat flakes, bran, oats, sultanas, raisins, currants, dried fruits and nuts to give you the energy to sustain you throughout the day? Add some fresh fruit or natural yoghurt to supply the necessary vitamins and minerals. Eat wholemeal toast for your fibre and have skimmed milk or fruit juice on your muesli. Instead of tea or coffee (both high in the toxin caffeine) try a herbal infusion.

By eating a good breakfast which releases energy throughout the day you can wave goodbye to the snacks which you may otherwise be tempted to eat mid-morning. Many of these snacks are 'empty' calories containing sugar, giving you a high boost of energy only lasting for about half an hour – just two chocolate biscuits will amount to about 300 calories. Better to choose a stick of celery, an orange or an apple which, while similar in calorie content, have the advantage of being complex natural foods to give you energy throughout the day.

Always read the labels on prepared foods. For example, tomatoes are a rich source of vitamins and low in calories (4 per ounce) *but* commercially prepared tomato ketchup with added sugar contains 30 calories per ounce. Sugar is simply 'empty' calories containing no nutrients, no minerals, no fibre, no protein, no vitamins. It makes us fat and rots our teeth. Cutting back on sugar is the easiest way to safely lose weight.

But some habits formed in childhood are difficult to get out of, as anyone with a sweet tooth knows. With determination one can gradually lessen the amount of sugar consumed (although really it is best cut it out altogether). If you must drink tea or coffee, try it unsweetened. If you find it difficult have weak tea or coffee and accompany it with an apple or a glass of water to enhance its flavour and dispel the craving. What seems impossible is worth pursuing in the knowledge that pounds will soon drop off through the dramatic decrease in calorie intake. Once the habit is broken it's surprising how the smallest amount of sugar will taste sickly and horrible. Look for tinned fruit in natural juice instead of syrup. And choose low calorie soft drinks and unsweetened fruit juices. Sweets, chocolates, cakes and biscuits just have to go. If all else fails to satisfy the sweet tooth then at least use a sugar substitute in cooking and in drinks. Saccharin is one of the many excellent sweeteners on the market. It could save you five teaspoonfuls of sugar which can be found in an ordinary soft drink.

As careful as you may be selecting your food, adding sauce, gravy, custard or cream will bump up the calorie content of the meal dramatically. To keep the calorie content low when eating salad, use natural yoghurt as a dressing or low calorie salad dressing. Eat your fruit fresh; there are 35 calories in one portion of fresh peaches but the same portion canned, in syrup, contains 100.

There's nothing nicer than having a meal out in a restaurant but once again choose your food with care. Avoid foods cooked in rich creams and sauces. Cut off excess fat from meat which you should eat grilled, not fried. A chicken breast contains approximately 450 calories but if the skin containing the fat is removed it will contain less than 350 calories. Generally, fish dishes have a lower calorie content than meat dishes and are a slimmer's friend. They will help to keep cellulite at bay by controlling weight gain. But avoid *all* fried food. Fresh boiled potatoes are delicious but mash them with butter and the calorie content increases; bake them around a roast in the oven and the calorie content gets higher; slice them and deep fry them as chips and they are just full of fat; when a potato is sliced very thin and deep fried it becomes the delicious crisp which is loaded with excess calories! And, still on the subject of snacks, watch out for the innocent looking peanut, especially the salted variety – there are 160 calories per ounce of peanuts! And by the time these have been processed into peanut oil they will contain 255 calories per ounce.

Sandwiches can be effective against cellulite if made with wholemeal bread and a low calorie butter substitute. Filled with tuna and cucumber, or cottage cheese and celery, for example, they can be healthy and nutritious, especially when they are accompanied by fresh fruit and yoghurt.

Your fight against cellulite is helped by careful shopping and buying foods to control weight gain, provide nutrition, avoid the accumulation of toxins and cut out excess fluid retention. Many of the ingredients for healthier eating can be found in any supermarket or greengrocer. The range of fruit and vegetables is endless with fresh local produce and colourful, exotic foods from countries throughout the world. Many are packed with the vitamins and minerals essential to good health and are best prepared and eaten raw. If you do cook them use the minimum amount of water and don't add fat.

Bright green and orange vegetables are the most nutritious. These include spinach, kale, sprouts, cabbage, broccoli, green peppers, lettuce, carrots and tomatoes. Potatoes (particularly when cooked in their skins), and also turnips, are excellent nutritionally. Citrus fruits such as oranges, lemons and grapefruits are full of vitamin C as are peaches, melons, pineapples and apricots. Fruits such as strawberries, blackberries and blackcurrants are excellent and nutritious. Our bodies need about five servings of fruit and vegetables a day, each serving consisting of about one cup's worth.

Butter, cream and many cheeses have a high fat content and their calories soon pile on those extra pounds thus encouraging cellulite. Many of these foods, which are unnecessary from a nutritional point of view, can be replaced by products with a lower fat content which are no less delicious once the taste buds have been re-educated. Butter can be replaced by low-fat spreads, and lard by vegetable cooking oils. Skimmed milk should be bought instead of full fat milk, and once again the useful yoghurt can serve as a substitute for cream. Plain cottage cheese has the lowest calorie content (25 calories per ounce). Gruyère and Stilton Blue cheese top the list with 130 calories per ounce, followed by Parmesan, cream cheese, Cheddar and Cheshire all at 120. Edam and Camembert with 85 calories each per ounce are a happy compromise but cottage cheese with 25 calories per ounce is the best aid to calorie counting! Eggs complete the list of dairy products which play a valuable part in our daily dietary needs.

For those living life in the fast lane with little time for the culinary arts, modern technology has come to the rescue with the increase in exciting ready-made frozen dishes. The variety of these is on the increase daily, and they are quick and easy to cook. They provide instant meals with the added advantage of having their calories and ingredients marked clearly on the side of the packet.

Many quality restaurants have led the way in the last few years to more sensible eating by making formal meals lighter and less rich; *nouvelle cuisine*, for example, is well appreciated by today's dietitians. It has caught on and has also become the basis for many recipes for today's busy housewife. With the careful use of herbs and seasonings even the most humble vegetable or most simple of fish can become true taste sensations. These recipes use less sauces and more fresh products steamed or cooked with only the slightest hint of butter, olive oil and lemon juice. It's a simple but healthy way to cook. And, as I mentioned before, it is essential to drink plenty of water to help wash out the system.

To help beat cellulite, special diets have been devised. I've included one which seems to me to be particularly good. However, because it isn't always practicable to follow a special diet, simply learning more about our dietary needs is time well spent.

Recommended Anti-Cellulite Diet

This is a diet aimed at balancing natural foods, vegetable juice and herbal infusions. The purpose is to cleanse the body of initial impurities and it should not be followed for more than three days without consulting your doctor.

ON WAKING
A glass of hot water with the juice of half a lemon.

BREAKFAST
(to be taken 20 minutes after the initial drink)
⅓ each of cucumber, beetroot and carrot juice (the cucumber acts as a diuretic to take away excess water; the other two vegetables give energy and vitamins). Fresh fruit salad – any fruits *except* banana.

LUNCH
A large glass of the same vegetable juice.

DINNER
1 sliced ripe tomato, topped with lemon juice and a drop of oil, a touch of sea-salt and basil or marjoram for flavouring. (A small quantity of oil *is* necessary because certain vitamins and minerals cannot be absorbed without it.) 2 steamed, non-starch vegetables (e.g. string beans, cabbage, carrots, parsnips, turnips, courgettes or celery, with a very little butter).

BEDTIME
1 glass of vegetable juice.

DRINKS
A herbal tea containing an infusion of equal parts of couch grass roots and peppermint.

Finding the Formula

A healthy diet should be sensible, well balanced and made up of the following formula: four portions of carbohydrate, two portions of protein and one portion of fat. Let's take a closer look and discover in which foods these essential ingredients are to be found.

Carbohydrates

Carbohydrates are our best source of energy. The recommended minimum dietary requirement is approximately 30g of carbohydrates each day. These can be found in cereals, vegetables, fruits, sugars, starches and alcohol. However, it's essential not to have all four daily portions of carbohydrates at one time. They shouldn't be eaten together at the same meal but should be spread out throughout the day to provide us with constant energy.

Many vegetables are full of fibre (which isn't lost through cooking). Fibre helps the digestive tract with bulk and roughage to ensure an efficient digestive system. Foods rich in fibre are often low in fats and sugars and carry a lot of water. They fill you up but since their calorific content can be negligible they are advantageous when calorie counting. They can also be very satisfying. For example, it takes roughly ten times as long to absorb a certain number of calories found, for instance, in a whole apple as to absorb the same number in the form of a glass of apple juice.

All cereals provide good quantities of natural fibres and sugars. These are absorbed slowly by the body and help to stabilize the sugar level of the blood. Fibre is found only in foods that grow from the ground; animal products do not contain it. Our bodies need 30g of fibre each day. Dried beans are a rich source but need careful cooking – soak them overnight then throw away the water and boil the beans for at least ten minutes. They can be used in stews, soups or cold in salad meat or fish dishes. Jacket potatoes and whole-meal bread are nutritious and rich sources of fibre.

Proteins

Proteins are indispensable in the formation of a strong body and in the maintenance and repair of body tissue. They are also important in combating the ageing effect that cellulite has on the skin. A balance between animal protein and vegetable protein is the ideal to aim for. The body does not differentiate between proteins, whether they be meat, fish, milk, cheese, eggs, vegetable or cereal. However, if you choose meat it must be lean and you must always cut off excess fat from bacon, roasts and all meats in general. It is preferable to buy fish or chicken which contain less calories than red meat, and grill, steam or bake. If you do fry foods use a non-stick pan which requires little or no fat at all. Under no circumstances must protein be done away with.

A lack of protein will result in muscle waste and premature ageing of the skin. In order to calculate a daily ration of protein it should be remembered that one 100g of meat or fish provides 20g of protein; one litre of milk provides 36g; a yoghurt provides 4g and an egg 6g. 100–120g of meat or an equivalent choice from the protein list above is sufficient for your daily quota.

Fats

Basically there are two types of fat: saturated and unsaturated. The saturated fats are found in beef, lamb, pork, suet, lard and dripping as well as in dairy produce such as milk, butter and cheese. They can also be found in coconut and palm oil, chocolate, cooking fat, hard margarine, cakes, biscuits, sauces and puddings. Saturated fats are linked with cholesterol and with a higher risk of heart disease as well as obesity.

Poly-unsaturated fats are found in vegetable oils, soft margarine and in nuts and oily fish and are infinitely preferable to the saturated variety.

Try to cut down on animal fats by choosing low-fat spreads, and use soft rather than ordinary margarines. A healthy adult does not need more than about 5g of fat a day.

The majority of fats are absorbed and passed into the living cells where they remain an important energy reserve. But excess fat soon forms unwanted and unsightly stores on our body where we least want them. This can happen all too easily if there is an imbalance between the food we eat and the food our bodies need and too much fat makes us overweight and blocks our arteries. It's very important to help yourself prevent cellulite by eating less saturated fats.

Some fatty products are easily recognizable by their colour: the white, cream, yellow and gold of cream, butter, oil and margarine, for example. Because butter and cream are rich in saturated fats they can contribute to the blocking of the arteries. Margarines which contain sunflower and other oils rich in unsaturated fats may be eaten safely in larger amounts. So if, like me, you can't do without butter (part of my West Country upbringing), keep it only for breakfast time on wholemeal toast and try to use margarines and low-fat spreads for all your other cooking and sandwiches.

Cheeses are a rich source of fat and along with other milk products are also our principal source of calcium, essential to the building of strong bones and teeth. One or two yoghurts a day (low-fat of course), plus 50g of cheese will provide us with the necessary calcium. If preferred, choose any low-fat cheese from the extensive range available from shops and supermarkets but be sure to select carefully. There are even some yoghurts and white cheeses containing 0% fat and these are marvellous to use in homemade sauces and soups.

Mineral salts, trace elements and vitamins are also required to maintain a balanced diet. These are of benefit to the bones, blood and nerves. They are found in abundance in fresh green vegetables which should be eaten twice daily, preferably raw. Only a little water should be used when cooking them or better still they should be steamed so as not to destroy the mineral and vitamin content. The water used in cooking vegetables shouldn't be wasted but conserved and made into healthy soups and sauces. Let's take a closer look at the principal minerals, trace elements and vitamins required by the body.

Minerals

Phosphorous is needed for teeth and bones. It is found principally in cheese, fish, meat, eggs, nuts and cocoa.

Calcium, which we have talked about before and which works with vitamin D to build teeth and nails, is essential for bone growth and maintenance. It is found in all dairy products such as milk, cheese, yoghurt. Found also in small whole fish, like sardines, and in smaller quantities in nuts, pulses and bread.

Potassium is important for muscle tissue, it helps in relaxation and converts sugar into energy. It is required to balance body fluids. It is supplied by foods such as meat, fish, wholegrains, wheat germ, bran, nuts, potatoes, vegetables and salads.

Magnesium is an important constituent of the bone and helps nerve and muscle functioning. It can be found in bread, rice, cereals, vegetables, and many nuts including hazelnuts.

Sodium is an important constituent of blood, bones and body fluids. This is found naturally in all fresh foods and in salted meats, fish, shell fish and processed cheese.

Trace Elements

These are the metals and other elements that are regularly present in the tissues and they are known to be essential for normal metabolism.

Iron is essential for red blood cell formation. Foods rich in iron are liver, kidney, heart, game, shell fish, dried fruits and vegetables, beans, pulses and spinach. Tiredness, lethargy and anaemia are all symptoms of possible iron deficiency.

Copper is essential in the formation of the red blood cells and helps to keep calcium in the bones. It is present in liver, shell fish, nuts, pulses, dried fruit and green vegetables.

Iodine is needed by the thyroid gland to enable it to function correctly. Fish, sea food, sea weed and iodized salt are valuable sources. It is recommended as part of an anti-cellulite diet for its diuretic properties.

Small amounts of **manganese**, **chrome** and **zinc** are also necessary for normal body function and the required levels are usually present in a sensible balanced diet. Zinc helps improve immunity against disease.

Vitamins

A cocktail of vitamins in the form of pills is available in neat little pots and boxes from chemists and health food stores. Yet everything we eat contains vitamins and it's actually questionable whether we need to take supplements of any of them. If you are in doubt as to whether your diet is deficient in one or several vitamins then the doctor is the person to consult for advice.

Let's pause for a moment to look more closely at who could be at risk from vitamin and mineral deficiency. Firstly, people who don't eat a balanced diet. Their eating habits are bad; they eat snack or junk food and not enough fresh and natural food. The diet contains too much processed and refined food.

Secondly, anyone who has been seriously ill or who is recovering from an operation, as well as women who take the contraceptive pill or use diuretic tablets.

Also at risk are those people with poor digestion or those who take an excessive number of laxatives which cause the food to pass through the gut too quickly to allow absorption of vitamins and minerals from the food.

Strict vegetarians or those on a weight controlled diet may be at risk, too, since they may suffer from a deficiency of essential nutrients.

We ought now to take a closer look at the more important vitamins, to see what they do and where they can be found naturally.

Vitamin A is essential for growth and is important in maintaining healthy eyes. It is to be found in milk, butter, eggs, margarine, fish (such as herring and fish liver oils) and liver. Also it is in green and yellow vegetables and fruits, such as broccoli, apricots and carrots. (Yes, there is some truth in the old wives' tale that eating carrots helps you to see better in the dark!)

The **B group of vitamins** (B_1, B_2, B_3, B_5, B_6 and B_{12}) assist in the regulation of the nervous system, the formation of red blood cells, the metabolism and they help give us our energy. They are present in meat, especially liver and kidney, fish, cereals (in particular, whole grain cereals), green vegetables, dried vegetables (such as beans), potatoes, milk, cheese and nuts.

Vitamin C is possibly the most important vitamin of all. It helps give us our energy and is important in the formation of collagen, the substance in our skin which helps wounds to heal. It provides a resistance to viral and bacterial infections and keeps us free from everyday coughs, colds and 'flu. It can be found in all citrus fruits and green vegetables and most particularly in blackcurrants and rose-hips.

Vitamin D is important for the health of our bones and teeth. Foods rich in this vitamin include fish (particularly oily fish), liver, margarine (less in butter) and egg yolk. Vitamin D is also formed in our skin when exposed to sunlight.

Vitamin E is concerned with the general maintenance of the body and as the years go by it can assist in preservation and the anti-ageing process. It can be found in wheat germ, wholemeal bread, vegetable oils, eggs and nuts.

We all know that good health isn't automatic, so it's vital that we are aware of how to maintain it with the passing of the years. It's up to us to look after and make the most of ourselves. In doing so we can keep ourselves out of the doctor's already overcrowded surgery and live our lives to the full. So let's plan and think positive.

Remember, a sensible well-balanced intake of food is essential if one is to get the necessary calories (energy) to cope with the stress and strain of everyday life. Two thousand calories consumed in one sitting is going to make us fat but if they are spread throughout a busy day this should be the perfect amount needed to maintain a healthy body. However, if a weight loss is required our calorie intake should be less.

Any changes must be made gradually: my personal rule in order to maintain a well-balanced and varied diet is moderation in all things. Instant dramatic weight loss must be avoided since a sudden change in habits can be physically dangerous and disturb the equilibrium of the body. Prolonged adherence to 'fad' diets may result in the slimmers' disease anorexia or bulimia nervosa.

Time for Action

Make a positive start by keeping a list of all the food consumed every day. Write down everything eaten *or* drunk from your first waking moment until you clamber back into bed at night. This should be done for a whole week and it's essential not to cheat or miss anything consumed however small or innocent it may seem.

Next, analyse the various times during the day or night when more energy is required. Sometimes, at the weekends in particular, there will be changes in your dietary requirements as a result of a different level of activity to that which your body is used to.

The results of your analysis should prove fascinating. Examine them carefully, noting particularly when the energy level is at its lowest. That's the time when a boost is required to lift it up again enabling you to go on. When meal times and dietary content are designed to coincide with these 'lows', the result is a balance of your energy input and the energy expelled. When the correct balance is eventually found and adhered to, sensible eating becomes a pleasure and not a problem. If the new rules are obeyed then after just a few months the ideal body weight will eventually be found and will remain stable.

While you try to rid yourselves of extra pounds and cellulite you have only to change your eating habits slightly in order to reduce the calorie intake, an excess of which is causing the problem.

Salt encourages fluid retention so cut out processed foods, such as sausages, bacon, smoked and pickled foods, salted nuts and crisps. Very simply you can cheer up your cooking with herbs and spices which will help cut out the salt you may otherwise be

Are you a healthy weight?

Take a straight line across from your height (without shoes) and a line up from your weight (without clothes). Put a mark where the two lines meet.

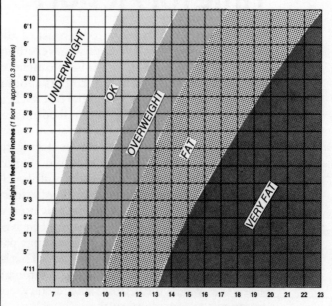

Your weight in stones *(1 pound = approx 0.45 kilograms)*

UNDERWEIGHT Maybe you need to eat a bit more. But go for well-balanced nutritious foods and don't just fill up on fatty and sugary foods. If you're *very* underweight, see your doctor about it.

OK You're eating the right *quantity* of food but you need to be sure that you're getting a healthy *balance* in your diet.

OVERWEIGHT You should try to lose weight.

FAT You need to lose weight.

VERY FAT You urgently need to lose weight. You would do well to see your doctor, who might refer you to a dietitian.

tempted to use to add 'taste'. Why not grow your own herbs (gardening is good exercise)? If you don't have a garden, a tub on a balcony or patio or even a window box will suffice. Experiment by cooking fish with parsley or fennel. Salmon cooked with dill is particularly delicious, as is tarragon and sage with chicken. Basil makes a tomato and cheese dish taste good, as does coriander used to season aubergines. One of my favourite dishes is using mint with cucumber and yoghurt.

Salads needn't be boring and if you have a garden you can grow your own lettuce, tomatoes, radishes, etc. Buy some sprouting beans, seeds and grains in your local health shop and leave them to sprout for three to six days. They're full of vitamins B and C and add a crisp crunch to any salad, as do nuts (chopped or whole) and red and white cabbage. Why not slice up button mushrooms, celery, and add spinach and fresh garden peas and young beans, or peas still in their pods? Add fennel, chives and fresh herbs for taste and for colour add fruit peeled and sliced such as oranges, grapefruit, peaches, apples or pears. The more exotic fruits, such as kiwi fruits, pawpaw, water melon and ordinary melons, add colour and taste. Lemon juice squeezed over the sliced apples will prevent browning and add taste. (Avocado pears should be used sparingly since they are high in calories and could add to your cellulite problem.)

Even when you're in a hurry or too tired to cook a proper meal you can still help yourself to a simple healthy snack, which will control your weight and prevent cellulite forming.

Baked beans on wholemeal toast can be nutritious, as are jacket potatoes filled with cottage cheese or yoghurt and chives. Wholemeal spaghetti is easy to make and delicious with a home made tomato sauce flavoured with herbs and spices. Sardines or pilchards (in tomato, not oil) are easily prepared, grilled on wholemeal toast. Or why not open a tin of tuna (in brine, not oil) and serve it with rings of tomato and onion on a bed of previously soaked and cooked butter and kidney beans. These are just a few very simple suggestions which may help to improve the infamous bottom line.

Eating Out

If you are eating out in a restaurant study the menu carefully and plan what you're going to eat from start to finish. Be sensible; begin with a fruit or vegetable starter and then you can spoil yourself later with a dessert. Conversely, if your starter is naughty but nice, finish your meal with a piece of fruit.

- For your main course avoid all fried foods whether meat, poultry, fish or vegetable. Instead choose something grilled, steamed or baked. As an alternative why not choose shell fish, pasta or rice. But beware of dressings, sauces, gravies and mayonnaise since these are often rich and full of calories. To accompany your meal eat plenty of fresh vegetables or opt for a side salad (ask for dressing to be served to you separately).

- Instead of gateau or ice cream decide on fresh fruit or a sorbet and choose your cheese with care. As a general rule remember the harder the cheeses the greater the calories.

- Throughout your meal drink either mineral water, fresh fruit juice or white wine which is low in calories.

- Finally, ask for decaffeinated coffee with skimmed milk and artificial sweeteners instead of sugar or cream.

Feeding Your Skin

Problem skin as well as excess weight will be encouraged to disappear if you cut out sugar, fat and processed foods. Fruit and vegetables rich in vitamins and minerals will nourish the skin, while the vitamin content will prevent the skin from ageing and also aid circulation thus preventing the formation of cellulite. The high fibre content of these foods, plus the water they contain, will flush out the system and prevent constipation.

Make your own natural fruit juices by freshly squeezing fruits which are full of vitamins and minerals. Drink them immediately though, before the vitamin C diminishes. They will cleanse the body and get rid of impurities and toxins, helping to improve the health and look of your skin and hair. Vegetable juices such as celery, watercress, carrots and beetroot can also help fight cellulite through their diuretic effects.

As we have seen, it is not food alone, however, that keeps our bodies strong and healthy. Exercise is important too. Sensible diet and simple exercise go together like hand and glove. Looking and feeling good encourages us to face the world, to take up the challenge of new activities and have the confidence to meet and make new friends.

Part 5

Dressing Hints

The Changing Face of Fashion

Over the ages fashions in clothing have changed. Since the First World War, women have fought for freedom and liberation which has expressed itself in, amongst other things, lighter clothing and a more fluid body line. Twentieth-century fashion designers have pampered us, giving us garments to work and play in, expressing our personalities and moods. They have released us from conformity, giving us practicality and freedom of movement.

Slimness has become a symbol of today's youth and beauty. Sensible eating, good physical appearance and a unisex approach to work and play have created the need to think slim. Unisex clothes such as trousers and sweat shirts which need firm thighs and a flat stomach complete the picture. Women in the sixties began to change their style by adopting trousers in preference to skirts, mens' shirts to pretty blouses, and trouser suits and blazers rather than figure-hugging dresses. Jeans became everyday wear and have remained so, even for the older age group. Jeans epitomize an adolescent figure by slimming the thighs, buttocks and stomach.

More recently we have witnessed the increased popularity of the track or jogging suit, worn for comfort and ease of living. Flat boots, shoes or sneakers enable us to walk and run with safety. And we do, with longer, more determined strides and a lively gait. Our confident appearance is completed with shorter cropped hair, clean and fresh, swinging free, released from the tightly coiffed or pinned back styles of days gone by.

But let's just take a look at how dressing correctly can, perhaps, succeed where dieting may have failed.

Many women, however hard they try to improve their shape, will still be heavier on their bottoms than their tops. This is familiar in Britain where the traditional womanly shape is often bottom heavy, or 'pear shaped', while many Latin ladies in comparison are top heavy, with slim hips and big busts.

But never fear because once again help is at hand: the first rule is to be honest about our shape and proportions. The second is to take pride in our good points and to be realistic about our faults, making the most of the former, while minimizing the latter. And finally we must decide on our own style and not just follow fashion for fashion's sake.

Underwear

An important start can be made by wearing the correct underwear and buying the right size. Not everyone will see you in your bra and pants but that shouldn't mean buying and wearing just any old thing without proper fitting. As with any other garment the size stated on the label of an item of underwear doesn't always necessarily coincide with your exact measurements. So don't just guess at your bra size – try on different styles, avoiding straps which cut, cups which are too small or which leave you sagging. There are designs to suit everyone and it only takes a little more effort to find the right fit. It will be time and money well spent. Having selected your perfect bra, buy several of the same style so that you can wash and wear economically and conveniently.

When exercising it's important to support your breasts which have only the pectoral muscle for self-help. Discomfort can be felt by the small breasted, never mind the well endowed, while jogging or doing aerobics. There are many excellent specially designed sports bras in the shops which support, bend, and stretch comfortably with you whatever your sport.

As a result of our new-found freedom and sporty image corsets and girdles are becoming a thing of the past. Now that we know that we ourselves must control our curves through diet, exercise and slimming aids, we no longer depend on garments to bind and control our stomachs and bottoms with hooks, bones and elastic. But, should a little help be required, support tights are excellent. They control and relieve aching legs, support varicose veins and gently mould the thighs, bottom and tum'. There is an ever-increasing number of manufacturers producing tights of varying support which both feel and look good.

Hosiery manufacturers are also helping to improve the bottom line with their new 'panti-tights': fine denier tights for unblemished legs combined with a control panty all in one. They're great to wear with anything, even trousers, and they do away with the unsightly panty line which can so often spoil the look of an outfit.

A slim petticoat completes the picture by helping tops to hang better, creating a smoother line. All underwear needs to be washed regularly and given a final rinse in a fabric conditioner to prevent static which can cause garments to cling to and accentuate ugly bulges.

Fabrics

Certain fabrics are less kind than others and need to be watched out for when buying clothes. Knitted garments need careful choosing. Knitted wool jersey, jersey silk or lycra can cling tightly and look cheap (be doubly aware of static). If these are your favourite fabrics then buy a size too large – loose sweaters are better than tight ones to emphasize and add proportion to the top half. Blouses and shirts should be full and generous, perhaps with padded shoulders or puffed sleeves to help add to the illusion and detract from the hips. Polo-necked sweaters, especially mean cut ones, create a skinny effect. Better to choose a softer, draped cowl neck line instead. Choose tops made of fabrics with 'body' of their own which will help to create more shape, and avoid hard materials which don't mould and just look stiff.

Dressed to Kill

Colours are all important: have fun and enjoy colour and, as with every aspect of your clothing, use it to draw attention to your better points while playing down the bad ones. Colour co-ordinated tops and bottoms, whether skirts or trousers, can create a long sleek sophisticated look. If you are using various tones of one colour emphasize the good points with the lighter tone and detract from the bad points with the darker one.

A straight skirt in a good fabric can be slimming but, in a cheap fabric, can really show those inches. A gathered skirt in soft quality fabric can fall and flatter into folds whereas those same gathers in a harder fabric will poke out and seem to pile on the pounds.

Elasticated waistlines on skirts and trousers give added comfort as well as accommodating the loss of inches during and after your successful slimming.

Tailored trousers can be a problem to buy and need very careful selection. Darker colours as well as being practical will also be most effective in creating a more slender look. Jeans are an important part of the modern woman's wardrobe but as I mentioned earlier they can be bad for our all-important circulation if worn too tight. They can also act as the old-fashioned girdle did by giving the wearer a false sense of muscle tone with their constricting support. Far more flattering and comfortable to wear are the looser tracksuits or all-in-one flying suits which are acceptable and practical everyday garments. In the case of the tracksuit it pays to spend that little bit extra on a material which will hold its shape and which won't sag at the knees and bulge at the bottom.

Be cautious with patterns and prints. Once again use

their effect (as bold as you dare) to emphasize the good points drawing the eye away from the bad, where it's safer to use the plain fabrics to minimize size. Bright colours, patterns, prints, stripes and spots can be fun to wear if you are a confident enough character to carry them off. But as my mother used to say to me 'if in doubt, leave them out'. Good advice of which I have taken heed many a time; it's always better to err on the side of caution. Instead, use accessories to add a touch of flamboyance to your outfit. Brightly coloured scarves or interesting bags can draw attention away from the figure. A dramatic belt of an unusual colour or detail can focus attention on a small waistline which should be shown and not hidden. A piece of jewellery worn close to a pretty neck can emphasize a face or beautiful hair. And if your skin is smooth and you have good shoulders, why not bare them?

Even a less than perfect waistline ('perfect' being ideally eight inches smaller than the hips) need not be draped in baggy fashions in order to disguise a big bottom. Most department stores and clothes shops sell separates which can be matched up to form a complete outfit both parts of which can fit well producing an overall well-put-together look.

Finally, always be prepared to spend that little bit more when buying your clothes, particularly skirts and trousers. Good quality fabrics and a better cut cost more but the results are well worth it. Creasing doesn't enhance the look of trousers and a crumpled skirt will not look smart. Cheap and cheerful can always apply to fun clothes and accessories but invest wisely in basics.

Part 6

Conclusion

We have now discovered what cellulite is, how and where it forms. We are now also aware that it affects many women regardless of age, although the stage of life is crucial in determining the cause of action, as cellulite is a condition for which action *can* be taken.

As you will recall, cellulite is most likely to form at or around the ages of twelve or thirteen (in other words, around the time of puberty), during pregnancy, and on reaching the menopause. During the awkward stage of puberty and the onset of the menstrual cycle, the young adolescent girl searches for her identity and forms her character. In pregnancy the young woman's body undergoes fundamental changes which upset her both mentally and physically. The third stage, the menopause, brings about distinct body changes along with the cessation of menstruation. These three important milestones can result in stress, which can lead in turn to an uncontrolled diet, feeling of lethargy, and possible depression. However, this vicious cycle can be prevented by being aware of your own body and honestly recognizing your pitfalls, and combining it with sensible eating and a form of exercise which will both suit *you* and be therapeutic.

French women have for centuries taken care of and pride in their bodies. By contrast, women in Britain and many other countries have, until fairly recently, felt guilty about spending time and money on themselves. Pampering and listening to your body have only now become acceptable, and are slowly replacing the need to 'go for the burn'. As we have seen, a pleasurable massage with oil, cream or gel can aid both your mental state and your cellulite. Remember also that a healthy, balanced diet coupled with a gentle yet effective exercise programme need not be a chore. In short, your body *can*, if you wish it to, become a source of rest, relaxation and pleasure.

Finally, do not forget the importance of good dress sense, as clothes can both enhance and worsen your shape. Always dress to suit your particular figure, and don't wear unflattering clothing simply because a current fashion dictates that you should do so. Once more, individuality is the key.

This book has outlined some of the ways in which you can turn your wobbles into wiggles. After all, you owe it to yourself to look after your body, or maybe even to rediscover it! And if, at certain moments in life, your body mechanics break down and the bulge threatens to take over, don't give in – remedies *are* at hand to put them right.

So care for yourself and the shape you're in, and keep on keeping fit!

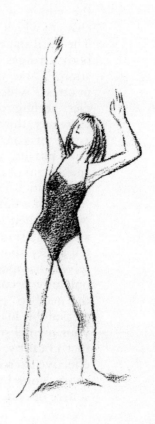

Questions & Answers

Q. **What is cellulite, who gets it and why?**

A. Cellulite is an abnormal accumulation of fat, toxins and fluids deposited in the skin, most commonly in the area around the bottom line. Any woman of any age or size can have cellulite. It can be caused by hormonal problems, circulatory problems, incorrect diet and lack of exercise.

Q. **How can you tell the difference between cellulite and ordinary fat?**

A. Press some of the flabby fat on the thigh or bottom with your thumb. If the print remains that is one sign. The skin may hurt if pinched and will look pitted like the peel of an orange. These are the three clinical signs of cellulite. Ordinary fat is by contrast spongy, smooth and doesn't hurt.

Q. **When does cellulite form?**

A. A large percentage of cellulite forms during the three stages of female development: at puberty, during pregnancy and in the pre-menopausal years.

Q. **Do men get cellulite?**

A. No, not generally, but very occasionally men who suffer from liver disease or who are undergoing hormone therapy get it on their stomachs and necks.

Q. **What can I do to help rid myself of cellulite?**

A. You must look at your lifestyle and make changes. You must improve your general health by learning to eat correctly and take more exercise. Massage and spot-reducing products can help.

Q. **If I diet and lose weight will the cellulite automatically disappear?**

A. Not necessarily; cellulite is very stubborn and often requires special attention. But take heart, there are many products in the shops which you yourself can use in your own home, or trained beauty therapists would always be pleased to assist you in beauty salons and clinics.

Q. **Do massage and exercise have any effect on cellulite?**

A. Exercise tones and strengthens your body as you lose weight. Massage works on cellulite spots by breaking down the nodules of fat thus improving the circulation and helping to disperse excess fluids and toxins. The preparations used in massage help soften and revitalize the skin.

Q. **How long will it be before I see a positive effect on my cellulite?**

A. To defeat your cellulite you would be advised to tackle several aspects of your lifestyle including diet and exercise as well as spot reducing. All of this takes time. However, an improvement should be seen after three weeks of spot-reducing treatment although it will be several months before the beneficial effects of improved diet and exercise are noticed. Once you've discovered the winning formula though, stick with it for life.

Q. **Is there any way I can disguise my heavy thighs and big bottom?**

A. Yes, clever dressing can make you appear slimmer. A darker skirt or trousers worn with a lighter top will minimize your hips (but don't wear either too tight). Colourful and interesting blouses and sweaters will attract the eye to the top and detract from your bottom. Tunic tops and sweaters and long jackets will help to disguise your bottom line.

Appendix 2

Glossary

Adipose tissue Tissue containing fat.

Calorie A measure of energy in food and drink.

Cellulite Subcutaneous fat alleged to resist dieting. Appears on women's thighs and bottoms in particular.

Cellulitis An acute inflammation of the skin. Not to be confused with cellulite.

Collagen The main protein constituent of white fibrous tissue (skin, tendon, bone, cartilage and all connective tissue).

Decongestant Agent which relieves or eliminates congestion.

Dermis The deep inner layer of the skin beneath the epidermis containing connective tissue blood vessels and fat.

Diuretics Substances which promote the secretion of urine.

Echotomograph A device that determines depth by measuring the time taken for a pulse of sound to reach an object and for the echo to return.

Epidermis The thin protective outer layer of the skin.

Gel A semi-rigid jelly like colloid (substance in a non-crystalline state) in which a liquid is dispersed in a solid.

Hypodermis The lower layer of the skin.

Lipid A fatlike substance existing in human tissue which is an important structural material in living organisms.

Lipolytic This causes the chemical disintegration or splitting of fat.

Liposuction Removal of fat by suction.

Lymphatic system An extensive network of capillary vessels that transports the interstitial fluid of the body as lymph to the venous blood circulation.

Massage Kneading or rubbing parts of the body to promote circulation, suppleness or relaxation.

Metabolism The sum total of the chemical processes that occur in living organisms resulting in growth, production of energy, elimination of waste etc.

Nutrients Serving as or providing nourishment.

Obesity The deposition of excessive fat around the body, particularly in the subcutaneous tissue.

Oedema Abnormal infiltration of tissues with fluid.

Oestrogen Any of several ovarian hormones that stimulate changes in the female reproductive organs, and promote development of female secondary sexual characteristics.

Progesterone A steroid hormone secreted mainly by the *corpus luteum* in the ovary that prepares and maintains the uterus for pregnancy.

Subcutaneous tissue The tissue beneath the skin.

Thalassotherapy Therapy relating to water and the sea.

Thermograph A type of thermometer that produces a continuous record of a fluctuating temperature.

Toxin Product of a bacteria that damages or kills cells.

Vein Any of the tubular vessels that convey oxygen depleted blood from the capillaries to the heart.

Venous Pertaining to the veins.

Vitamin Any of a group of substances that are essential in small quantities for the normal functioning of the metabolism. They cannot usually be synthesized by the body but they occur naturally in certain foods.

Index

93